The Metabolic Syndrome Diet

By

Lynne D M Noble

Independently published 2020

Contents

About the Author

Lynne Noble was born in 1953 in Huddersfield, West Yorkshire. From a very early age, Lynne showed an interest in nutrition and genetics avidly reading any books that she could get her hands on at the time.

Initially, Lynne studied orthopaedics but events led her to work with the elderly mentally infirm. Here, her interest in neurodegenerative disorders and pain syndromes developed.

Lynne undertook rigorous programmes of study, completing her Cert Ed., (FE) BSc (Hons) and Adv. Dip Education simultaneously before moving onto her M.Ed.

From there she took further demanding programmes in Human Nutrition, Pharmacology, Neuroscience, Genetics and Immunology. During this time, she was given many prestigious awards for her academic work. It was noted then that Lynne was not afraid of tackling difficult subjects.

She began her law degree but ill health prevented her from pursuing this. However, in this time, she moved from being a foster parent to adoptive parent.

She has been instrumental in setting up projects in the community for disadvantaged groups.

She is a member of the Guild of Health Writers and the British Union of Journalists.

Now retired, she lives with her husband in a historic Georgian riverside town in the West Midlands. She enjoys gardening, watching her husband bowling and researching.

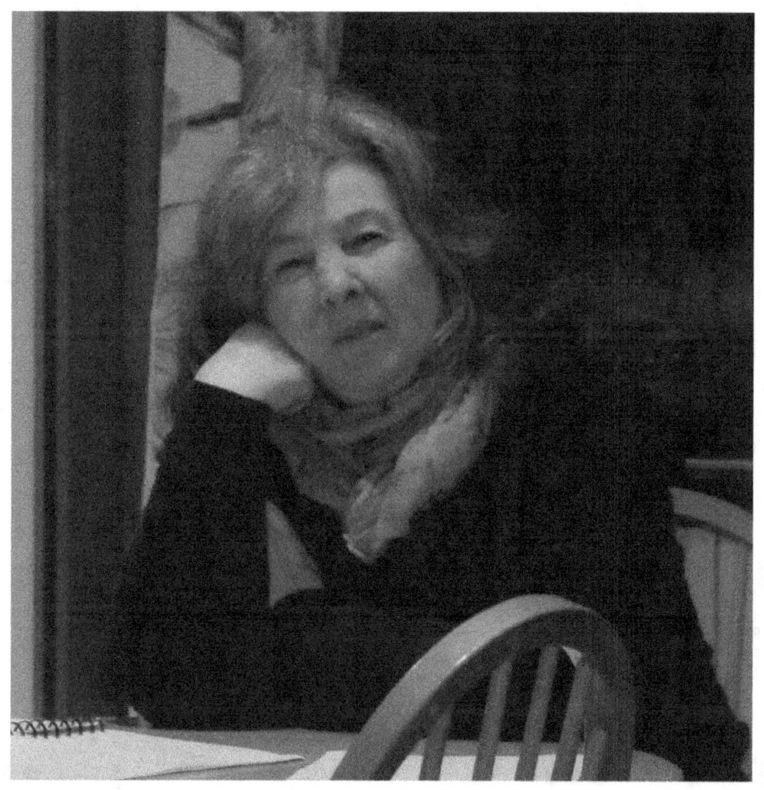

Author Lynne Noble at home

R H James, Illustrator Profile

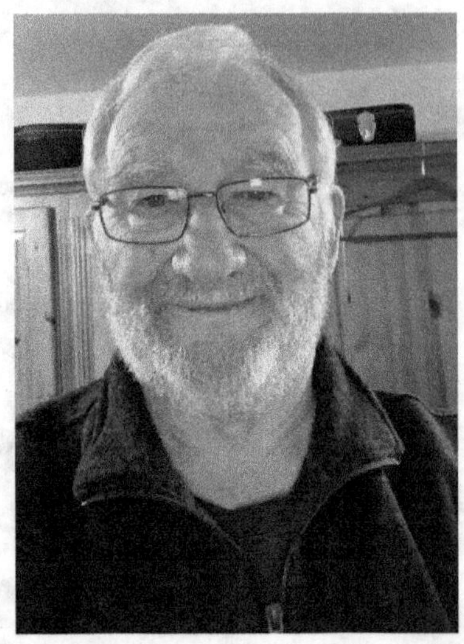

R H James or Bob as he likes to be known by, has been a keen doodler for many years although he has not been in print before.

Bob initially embarked on a career in agriculture and progressed to a career in teaching – particularly pupils with learning and behavioural difficulties.

In a voluntary capacity he has been involved in outdoor pursuit activities as a means of teaching young people

He was voluntary warden of a Mountain Centre in North Wales teaching life skills and improving confidence.

He has also been involved in working with scouts and is a Duke of Edinburgh assessor.

Preface

I hadn't seen my cousin for forty years. We had always got on well when we were children. As he was five years older than I, he took good care of me. When we finally caught up with each other, I was saddened to find out that he had diabetes, high blood pressure, abdominal obesity and high cholesterol levels.

His risk for stroke and heart attack was high.

He was insulin dependent and was on a wide range of medications to try and control the cluster of symptoms that he had.

Many of these had side effects and would have killed him in the end. One of his medications was a thiazide diuretic. Its mode of action is to get rid of allegedly excess fluid so that the heart doesn't have to work as hard, thus reducing blood pressure. This medication, apart from increasing urine flow, leaches potassium and magnesium at the same time.

Low magnesium and potassium levels are extremely concerning. Magnesium is required for over 300 actions in the body including lowering blood pressure, aiding sleep, allaying anxiety, maintaining fluid balance and alleviating constipation, balancing blood sugar among others.

Potassium is critical for many functions in the body. People who have low levels lose muscle mass, become brain fogged, feel tired, may have personality changes. They are likely to have bowel dysfunction in the form of chronic and seemingly intractable constipation. Potassium helps lower blood pressure and low levels will help form visceral fat and abdominal obesity.

I had just been commissioned to write a paper on metabolic syndrome and had already undertaken a great deal of research on the subject. The combination of this and my affection for my cousin, inspired me to write this book.

My cousin was in his seventies when we met. He had been attending a local slimming group for four years and not making much progress in reversing this syndrome.

With his determination and my professional skill combined, a new man is emerging. His blood sugars are stabilising; he has lost two stone. His blood pressure is responding to his weight loss. He says he feels better and he certainly looks much better.

BUT I doubt that he would have made it by himself. The GP had put him on medication after medication to control the cluster of symptoms that he had. This medication either made diabetes worse, increased blood pressure through various mechanisms or, in some cases, increased weight.

It appears to me that when someone presents with a symptom, that symptom - rather than the underlying cause - is treated. There are two things that are wrong with this approach.

Firstly, the patient is unlikely to ever stop taking the medication. Secondly, the side effects of the medication can make the medical condition worse in the long term.

One of the medications that my cousin was on had been documented at putting on an average of 10lb of weight.

My cousin was trying to lose weight in order to help his diabetes so this appeared particularly cruel and it didn't help his motivation or his diabetes.

If you are diagnosed with metabolic syndrome, it is particularly important that you do address it since it raises the risk of diabetes, stroke and heart disease.

This book will examine this syndrome and, just as importantly, how you can respond through diet to the particular difficulties this condition raises.

Diet is important but I am not a particular fan of counting calories or making meals time consuming or expensive. Most people do not have time for this nor do they have the money. It has to be easy and you have to understand the reasons why I recommend a particular course of action.

I will also look at common medications that are prescribed for metabolic syndrome and why they may be counter-productive. I will suggest dietary substitutes that don't have the dangerous side effects that are often prescribed for people with metabolic syndrome.

You will need:

- a good set of scales that do not change if you shift your weight on them. You will need to weigh yourself naked in the morning before you have breakfast.
- a blood pressure monitor
- a notebook so that you can monitor your results

You will keep a close eye on the changes in blood pressure, blood sugar (if you are diabetic) and log this in your notebook

You will initially need to log your waist circumference, painful though this may be.

You will also need to take a before photo and one every month thereafter.

If you have a smart phone, then there should be an app that you can download that logs how many steps that you take. For the first week the goal is to walk at least

2,000 steps but this should increase by one thousand at the beginning of every new week until you are up to 5000.

After that, try and increase by a further 500 steps every month. It's great if you can do more.

The aim is to get up to 8000 steps daily.

My cousin has an app that records his blood sugar levels and sends them directly to his smart phone. However, it doesn't record the other measurements that he needs to take.

You will find a system that works for you from this book. It will be a bespoke system that is relevant to your needs only. When you need to tweak it you will know how.

You may have noticed that certain things make it easier to lose weight but this goes against all the experts say.

You will read this book and think, 'Yes that applies to me.'

Could you be right? Well, yes you could. It is a lot easier losing weight eating chocolate than eating fruit for some people and there is good scientific evidence for this.

You will learn all this in this book.

Metabolic Syndrome – what is it?

Metabolic syndrome is a cluster of signs and symptoms that can be found together. They increase your risk for stroke, diabetes and heart disease. Approximately one in three adults in the UK and US have metabolic syndrome.

This cluster of conditions includes:

- high blood sugar
- high blood pressure
- raised low density lipoprotein – known as the 'bad' cholesterol
- high triglyceride levels
- fat laid down in and around the abdomen known as the 'apple shaped figure.'

The more of these conditions that you have the more you are likely to develop diabetes.

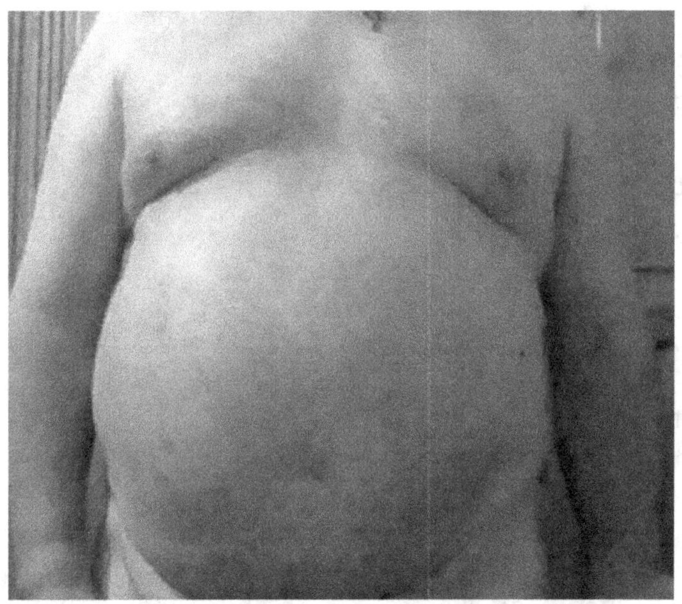

Apple shape, abdominal obesity associated with metabolic syndrome in 57-year old male.

Diabetes is becoming more and more common. One in sixteen people live with diabetes in the UK.

In the US approximately one in ten individuals are diabetic.

Diabetes is a systemic disease. This means it impacts every part of your body. Some of the conditions associated with diabetes are:

- loss of sight
- increasing risk of infection even with minor wounds
- nerve damage – pain or loss of sensation in the feet
- high blood pressure and increased risk of stroke
- kidney damage

Definitely one to be avoided at all costs.

How do we measure abdominal obesity to ascertain whether we have one of the conditions associated with metabolic syndrome?

For men a waistline of 40 inches or over and for women a waistline of 35 inches or over counts as abdominal obesity for the purposes of metabolic syndrome.

You don't need to go to a GP to have this measured. All you need is a simple measuring tape. Measure around the navel.

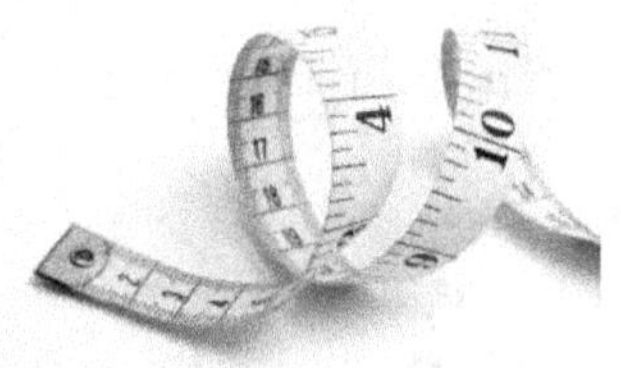

Measuring blood pressure is fairly easy. A sphygmometer can be bought from most good pharmacists. They are battery operated unlike the ones the doctors used to use when I was much younger. These were hand pumped and a stethoscope placed onto the skin to hear changes in sound that indicated the systolic and diastolic measurements.

The blood pressure always consists of two numbers. The higher number is known as the systolic and its 'normal' reading is 120.

The systolic reading occurs as the heart pumps blood through the arteries at high speed. If the arteries are relaxed and not clogged up, the blood will flow freely and unimpeded. The systolic will read 120.

If the arteries are semi blocked by plaque build ups, then the heart has to work harder to pump blood through the arteries. This will force the systolic to be higher.

Being overweight will increase the systolic purely because the blood volume and circulatory system will be greater. It follows then that the greater your body mass, the higher your blood pressure is likely to be.

The diastolic reading measures the blood vessels when dilated. That is, immediately after the heart has contracted (systolic reading) it relaxes producing a lower reading.

The text book diastolic is 80 so a 'perfect' reading is 120/80.

Some people believe that blood pressure will automatically go up as you age but this is not true. Raised blood pressure is a sign that something is not quite right. In needs investigating as the state of your blood pressure is a good indicator of your health.

However, most of the time, raised blood pressure is due to greater body mass index than the heart can cope with.

Low or average blood pressure is associated with good health.

It is quite possible to have low blood pressure and have a high waist circumference.

What we require are three of the conditions mentioned at the beginning of this chapter for a diagnosis of metabolic syndrome.

It is quite possible to have a waist circumference of over 35 inches for a woman but without the presence of two of the other conditions associated with metabolic syndrome you do not have it.

There are plenty of useful online charts – one of which is reproduced below – which can indicate whether you have cause to be concerned about your blood pressure readings.

When you take a blood pressure reading always take the reading from your right arm.

Make sure you are not stressed as this will artificially raise the reading.

Make sure that you have not eaten or drunk a hot drink as this will also raise the reading artificially,

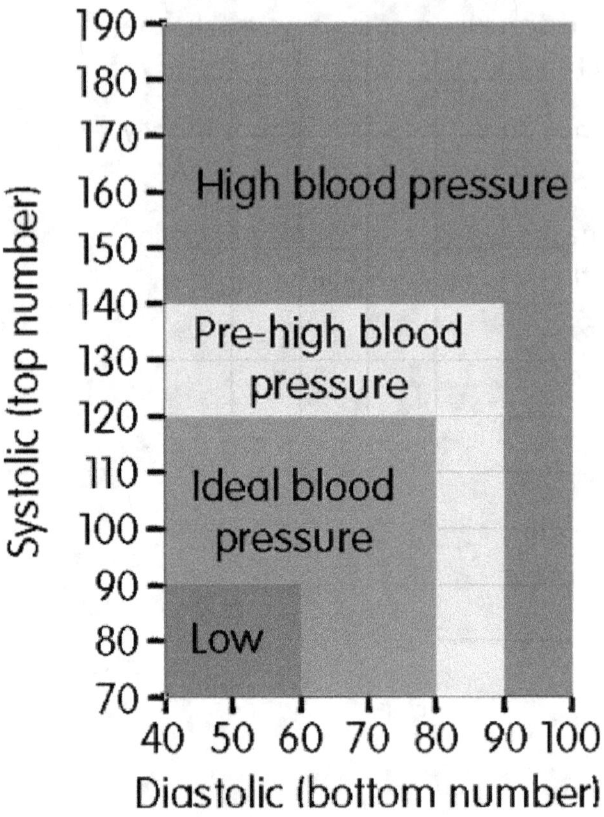

[1]Using this blood pressure chart: To work out what your blood pressure readings mean, just find your top number (systolic) on the left side of the blood pressure chart and read across, and your bottom number (diastolic) on the bottom of the blood pressure chart. Where the two meet is your blood pressure.

---

[1]

http://www.bloodpressureuk.org/BloodPressureandyou/Thebasics/Bloodpressurechart

Sit quietly for five minutes before taking the reading. Some GP's take three readings and use the average.

Only if the reading is very different from what you are expecting should you take another one after observing the above suggestions.

Steroid use and infection will raise blood pressure for their duration.

Now you should have measurements for your waist circumference and your blood pressure.

Although most people have a blood test for cholesterol levels taken at the surgery, there are some economically priced tests available online or in supermarkets.

The distinction between 'good' high density lipoprotein (HDL) and the 'bad' low density lipoprotein (LDL) is not as great as people are led to believe. The higher the LDL as you age, the better your memory is likely to be.

Nevertheless, raised cholesterol levels are one of the conditions associated with metabolic syndrome and so it is useful to know what acceptable levels are.

Cholesterol is reputed to combine with other substances such as calcium and contribute to blockages in the arteries, pushing up blood pressure.

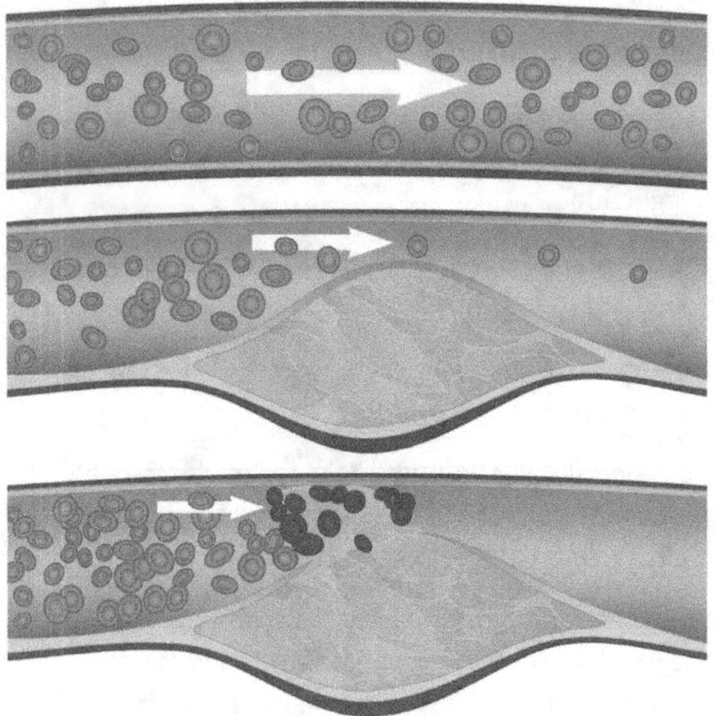

² cholesterol build up in arteries

² https://www.livescience.com/34712-ldl-cholesterol-buildup-causes-heart-attack.html

Total cholesterol

Below 5mmol/L	Desirable level
5 - 7.5mmol/L	Borderline to high risk
7.5mmol/L or higher	High risk

The chart above is perhaps a little too simplistic. It does not account for the fact that cholesterol has many benefits in the body including:

- making bile which helps with fat digestion
- is an integral part of all cells
- is required to make vitamin D from the sun's action on the skin
- has an important role in the composition of the outer coat of every nerve
- is needed to make an important brain chemical

and so on.

However, it is associated with metabolic syndrome.

If you have a cholesterol test at your GP surgery, then the amount of triglycerides will also be measured.

Triglycerides are a type of fat found in the blood. After you eat, any calories not needed at the time are converted into triglycerides and stored in fat cells.

Between meals, when this stored energy is required then hormones release triglycerides for this purpose.

It is easier using this energy immediately than storing and then releasing it which is why some gentle walking after a meal is so beneficial.

Now that we have an idea about what metabolic syndrome is we need to know how to reverse the condition.

Fortunately, the condition can be reversed although it is always harder to lose weight as you get older. Nevertheless, it is not impossible and there are plenty of things that you can do that will make the whole process easier. Calorie reduction will almost certainly reduce the amount of triglycerides in your system because triglycerides are excess energy which is not required at that time.

The health of the arteries can be improved too. It is fairly easy to lower cholesterol levels without the use of statins which have some damaging side effects.

It is my guess that most people will want to start with correcting abdominal obesity. So ..... you need to measure around your navel and log this measurement down.

Part of correcting abdominal obesity is examining the reasons why you overeat OR what foods you are eating that contribute to abdominal obesity.

As you will soon find out, not all calories are equal in spite of what is popular opinion.

It is important to reflect on this first.

Why do we eat three meals a day?

When three meals a day were the norm, people were involved in much heavier physical work. The typical English breakfast was meant to provide a manual worker with the energy to cope with long days using lots of muscle power.

Lunch time would probably consist of a ploughman's lunch with chunks of cheese and thick slices of wholemeal bread before an evening meal consisting of meat and two veg.

You will note that simple carbohydrates – those foods containing lots of sugar - or lacking fibre - did not exist in this diet.

This was a good diet because the lack of simple carbohydrates meant that insulin levels did not become excessively elevated.

 It is insulin that causes hunger and fat storage.

 It is insulin that makes you want to continue eating long after your nutritional needs have been satisfied.

Now breakfast may consist of:

- a muffin and fruit
- cereals and yogurt
- toast and jam
- a smoothie
- fruit

None of these are really all that healthy unless your cereal is wholemeal and the yogurt without sugar.

Fruit smoothies are notoriously high in fructose, a sugar that increases your blood sugar levels and insulin very quickly. They can lead to that slump that you feel after eating that causes you to doze off.

Fruit and cereal doesn't contain a great deal of protein.

 It is reaching your required amount of protein daily that stops you feeling hungry.

Much better high protein breakfasts are:

- eggs
- bacon
- whole meal sausage
- ham
- cheese
- wholemeal bread
- sugar free yogurt

- mushrooms
- *whole wheat cereal (All Bran)
- nuts

*Many whole wheat cereals tend to be carbohydrate heavy. This may make it quite difficult to maintain acceptable blood sugar levels although the fibre does help a little in maintaining them.

I found this out quite by chance when I embarked on my very first slimming diet and found that after I had eaten the recommended Weetabix, I was very hungry half an hour later.

I was investigating the glycaemic load of foods at the time. Out of curiosity, I looked up whole wheat cereals and found most of them would push blood sugar levels up quite dramatically.

The Glycaemic Index (GI) is a rating system from 0 to 100. It rates foods containing carbohydrates and shows how quickly that food would affect glucose levels if eaten on its own.

A low GI is anything less than a score of 55

An intermediate GI is a score that is found between 56-69

A high GI is a rating of between 70 and 100.

There are plenty of Glycaemic Index tables to be found on the internet but sometimes it is good to get an idea of foods and their glycaemic index value.

Table showing common foods and their glycaemic index value

Food	Glycaemic Index – approximate figures
White bread	75
Whole wheat bread	74
Boiled white rice	73
Boiled brown rice	68
Barley	28
Watermelon raw	78
Raw pineapple	59
Boiled potatoes	79
Rice crackers and crisps	87
Honey	61
Apple	36
Chocolate dark, milk	40 -45

Now there may be a few surprises with the above. Firstly, there is little difference between the GI of white or whole wheat bread.

Watermelon – touted as a very healthy food – is in fact very high on the GI. It may not contain fat but it will cause those blood sugar levels to rise and, as a result, insulin.

Rice crackers are also found to be very high on the GI, yet they are often advertised as being healthy because they are low in fat. Low in fat they are but when I tried rice cakes I found that they, too, made me feel very hungry shortly after eating them.

I did not have this problem with chocolate. Even though, at the time, I did not know which foods belonged where on the index, I could tell by how I felt shortly after eating them.

There are some great low sugar chocolate bars on the market that are no dearer than those normally bought that haven't reduced their sugar. Either though – whether low sugar or not - have major advantages over some fruits.

Sure, fruit doesn't contain fat but fat is not bad in sensible quantities. We need fat in our diet to absorb vitamins ADEK which are fat soluble.

These fat soluble vitamins are vital for our health and we would be sick very quickly without them.

In addition, fat slows down digestion and prevents a sugar spike so that extra insulin is not made.

If excess insulin is not made, then fat cannot be stored.

This is the principle on which the Atkins Diet works.

A chocolate bar with nuts makes a great snack when you are in a hurry or need something sweet. It is low on the glycaemic index because of the three types of fat in it.

These fats are good for good for you. They are:

- oleic acid – a monounsaturated fatty acid that helps to reduce inflammation
- stearic acid – a saturated fat (therefore it will not cause inflammation) that helps lower cholesterol
- palmitic acid – this is also a saturated fat. In **normal** quantities, this is a good fat as it is used for the composition of all cells.

We will look at the problems of too much palmitic acid later but it is sufficient to know at this point that some is necessary for normal metabolic purposes in the body.

Chocolate is made from the cocoa bean and, as such, is full of antioxidants. It is also full of the trace mineral magnesium.

Magnesium is involved in over 300 enzymatic reactions in the body including making sure that you don't retain water. It makes sure that the water balance in your body is just how it should be.

Magnesium keeps you calm, keeps your bowels moving, aids sleep and makes sure your bones are strong and healthy as well as having many more beneficial effects.

Magnesium is not the only beneficial nutrient to be found in chocolate and cocoa. Cocoa products contain a number of nutritional substances that help break down fat. In order to understand this, I am first going to explain a little about a substance found in many healthy foods that actually causes weight gain. It is called adenosine and it explains why exercise can be counter-productive when trying to lose weight.

Adenosine

**this chapter and the subsequent one is reproduced from
The Chocolate Diet and why it works**

Not many people have heard of adenosine never mind know what it does. However, it is an important nutritional substance when it comes to understanding why weight loss may not occur - even after rigorous dieting.

Adenosine is a regulatory molecule in metabolic processes. A metabolic process is a set of life supporting processes in an organism. They have one of three functions.

1. The conversion of food to energy so enable the basic functions of every cell.
2. The conversion of food to the basic building blocks for:

a) lipids which are fatty acids and glycerol.
b) protein which are amino acid
c) carbohydrates which are monosaccharides
d) nucleic acids which are nucleotides

3. The elimination of nitrogenous – or waste by-products –

Sometimes, the word metabolism refers to the total processes that allow the body to run efficiently.

Therefore, metabolic processes are vital for health.

In the brain, adenosine is a neurotransmitter (brain chemical that carries messages) that has an inhibitory action. It promotes sleep. Levels of adenosine rise throughout the day in response to exercise. This is an important concept that we shall return to shortly.

At the end of the day provided adenosine levels are high enough then arousal is suppressed and sleep promoted.

Adenosine has many other actions including energy metabolism and expenditure.

The more physical exercise that you do the more the more adenosine is produced. Adenosine helps muscles to adapt to exercise thus helping to prevent trauma. In addition, adenosine is also released in response to:

- Trauma of any kind
- Oxidative stress – where it helps to protect the brain
- Metabolic distress

Adenosine is found in all organs in the body where it has a diversity of functions including:

- Kidneys – decreased blood flow and decreased production of rennin from the kidney.
- Lungs – constriction of airways
- Liver – constriction of blood vessels and increased breakdown of glycogen to form glucose

- Heart – decreased heart rate and has antiplatelet action and increased diameter of blood vessels in peripheral organs.

Adenosine's numerous functions include:

- Relaxing vascular smooth muscle
- Regulating T cell proliferation and cytokine production - cytokines are small proteins that are secreted by cells of the immune system and have an effect on other cells.
- Relieving nerve pain including shingles
- **Inhibiting lipolysis**

Inhibiting lipolysis is the one that we are interested in.

Lipolysis is the breakdown of fat. Fats are broken down in our body by enzymes and water. Fat is actually stored energy and found in adipose tissue stores.

Fat has many uses including cushioning our bodies from trauma.

Excess calories – over and above our needs – are stored as triglycerides and broken down when we need the energy that is stored there.

This energy is useful in times of illness or when appetite is lost. The stored fat is broken down into fatty acids and glycerol providing an easily accessible form of fuel for the body.

Adenosine is used in the composition of adenosine triphosphate, also known as ATP.

ATP provides energy which is required to fuel many of the processes in living cells. For example, you cannot contract muscles without it or initiate nerve impulses.

The importance of ATP is demonstrated by its description of

The molecular unit of currency of intracellular energy transfer

Now ATP is synthesised from fatty acids and protein from lean meats - chicken and turkey, for example, and also from fatty fish and nuts. However, as adenosine inhibits lipolysis, eating these foods – including chicken and turkey – have to potential to increase weight gain through the inhibition of the breakdown of fat for fuel.

This may take some time to get your head around. We are so used to hearing that turkey and chicken are ideal foods for weight loss.

In some respects – within a calorie controlled diet - they may be. However, we cannot look at any food in the light of how many calories a portion contains. Any food has numerous nutritional substances contained within it and each of those will interact with an individual's genetic makeup and impact on many aspects of overall health.

Any of those other substances may promote or suppress weight gain. Currently, weight reducing diets have a tendency to restrict one of four factors:

- Carbohydrates
- Fat
- Protein
- Calories

However, there are many other nutrients in any food that may also have a bearing on an individual's body mass including adenosine.

Nevertheless, organisations or individuals, in the diet business, will address the dietary factor that is the simplest one to manage and further, will also maximise profits for them at the same time.

I also note that, as adenosine levels rise in response to exercise, then the breakdown for fat as a fuel is inhibited.

EXERCISE = GREATER PRODUCTION OF ADENOSINE = INHIBITION OF FAT BREAKDOWN FOR FUEL

This offers an explanation why exercise does not appear to be a good weight loss solution. Indeed, for many – including me – exercising actually appears to increase weight gain. Some of this may be due to increased appetite but, in the majority, it cannot be explained by this.

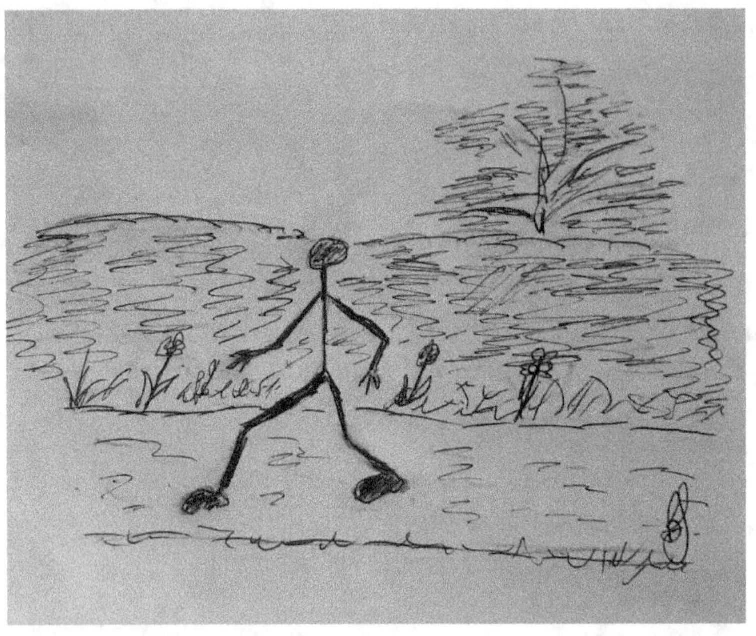

Exercise is useful for losing weight in some people but not for others

As adenosine containing foods are essential for energy transfer then we should not seek to limit them from our diet. However, we need to be aware that too many may – in genetically susceptible people – carry the risk for unwanted weight gain which is difficult to lose.

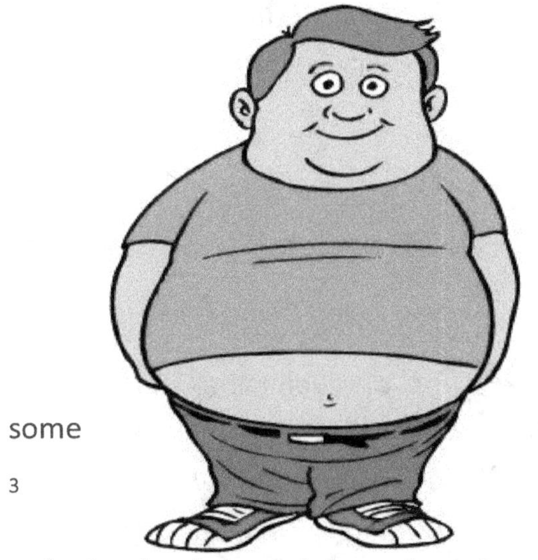

Reducing the amount of foods containing adenosine during calorie restriction would aid the breakdown of stored fat in some people.

3

reducing foods containing adenosine would enable the breakdown of stored fat for energy.

It may be that a diet that leans heavily towards lean meat may not always be the best diet for those who appear to be particularly susceptible to the effects of adenosine.

I know of many individuals who embark on a diet and find that they are utterly exhausted and failing to lose weight. Many of the foods that are recommended for calorie

---

3 https://www.clipart.email/clipart/fat-people-clipart-3171.html

restricted diets also contain the most amounts of adenosine. Therefore, the energy stored as triglycerides in fat cells, is not available to be used.

What are the main food sources of adenosine?

Adenosine is found in lean meats such as turkey and chicken, oily fish and nuts.

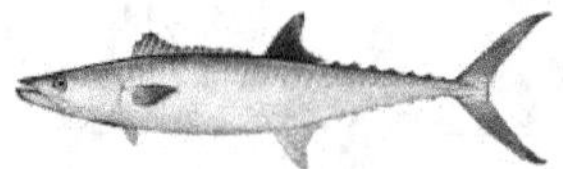

Mackerel contains good amounts of adenosine and therefore inhibits the breakdown of stored fat into a form that can be used for energy.

 However, we should not seek to exclude these foods from our diet as they contain many valuable nutrients. We merely need to reduce the amount of adenosine, in our diet, if our intake is high.

We could also block some of the adenosine from being taken up by the body.

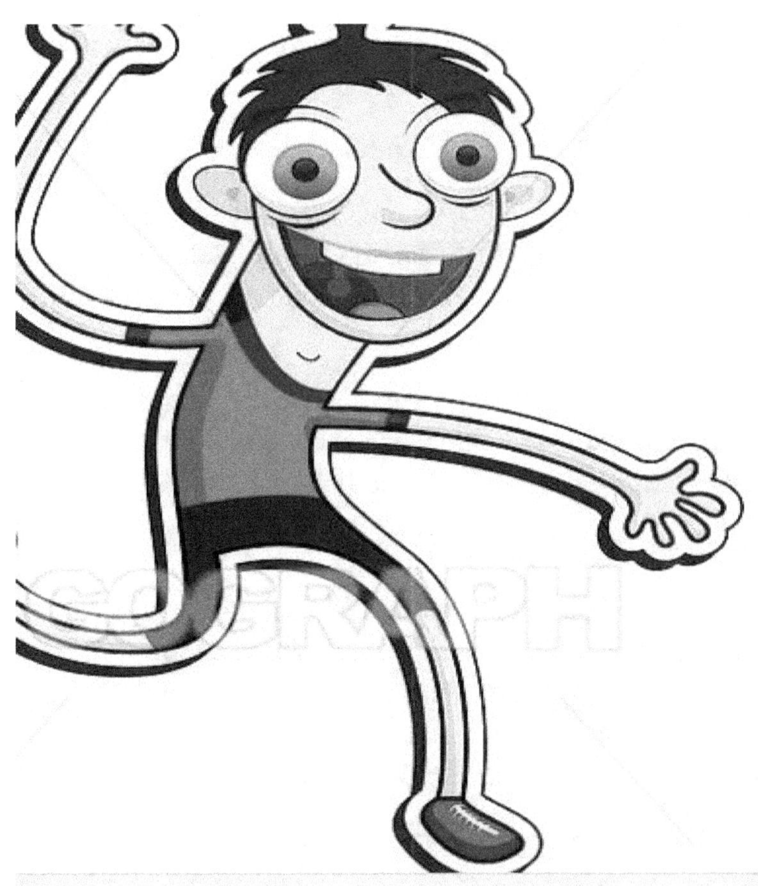

[4]Running increases the amount of adenosine in the body and inhibits the breakdown of fat.

It can be understood from the above that dietary recommendations which include lean meat, oily fish and

---

[4] gg56845818

exercise, actually inhibit lipolysis, the breakdown of fat stores for energy.

 It flies in the face of all we have been told.

When we have used the glucose that is immediately available for our needs, our hope is that calorie restriction and exercise will result in our fat stores being used for fuel, resulting in weight loss.

Clearly, this is not always the case. Adenosine is an explanation of why some individuals do not appear to be able to lose weight in spite of disciplined dieting.

What then can we do to block the effects of adenosine?

The answer lies in the methylxanthines – a group of substances that block adenosine receptors. Most people have never heard of methylxanthines but they will have undoubtedly eaten a common food stuff that contains one of the methylxanthines known as theophylline.

It is to the subject of theophylline that we now turn.

The Methylxanthines

Theophylline is a drug that is often used to treat respiratory disorders such as asthma and chronic obstructive pulmonary disease.

It helps to relax bronchioles enabling easier airflow through the respiratory tract.

It is also anti-inflammatory in action. However, for the purposes of the subject of this book, it is also an adenosine antagonist.

What exactly is meant by that?

On every cell there will be tiny receptors for adenosine. These receptors are specifically shaped to grab hold of adenosine and no other substance.

Sometimes, though, there are antagonists that can interfere with or inhibit the functioning of adenosine by blocking the receptors.

Theophylline interferes with the action of adenosine. It attaches itself to the adenosine receptors.

This action prevents adenosine from being able to bind to the receptors and inhibit the breakdown of fat into useable fuel for the body.

As one of adenosine's functions is to induce sleep, increasing theophylline in large amounts can cause insomnia.

Theophylline is found in tea (camellia sinensis) However, it is doubtful whether a nightly cup of tea contains enough theophylline to keep anyone awake.

Anyway, tea also contains theanine which induces calm and a feeling of all is well with the world.

 The main source of theophylline is cocoa. Dark chocolate which contains cocoa solids of 85% or upwards contains useful amounts of theophylline which acts as an adenosine antagonist.

 <u>Drinking cocoa or eating dark chocolate, high in cocoa solids, helps the breakdown of fat.</u>

Theophylline is not the only methylxanthine. As all methylxanthines have a role as antagonist of the adenosine receptors A_1 and A_2 then it is helpful if we look at some other common ones.

Caffeine and theobromine are the most abundant naturally occurring methylxanthines.

Theobromine – also found in cocoa – improves your circulation and respiratory system. It increases the activity of a cell called cyclic adenosine monophosphate (cAMP).

This messenger molecule activates an enzyme which reduces inflammation.

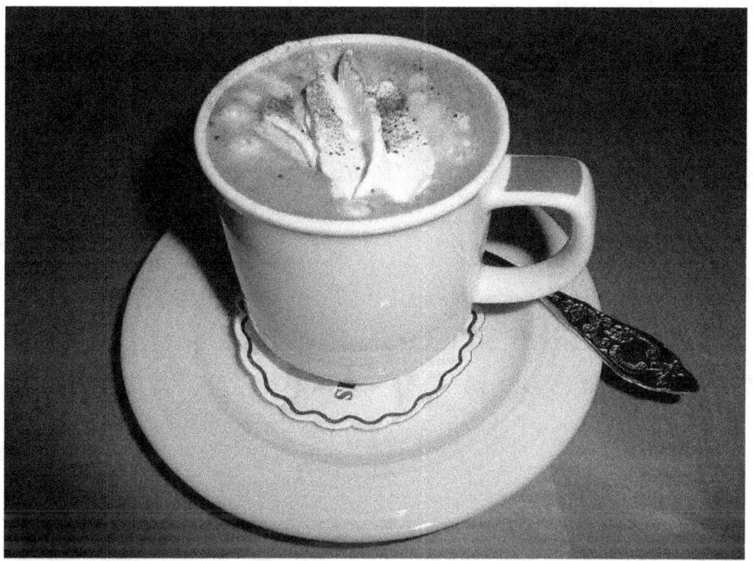

Cocoa can help with weight loss by the action of theophylline on adenosine receptors. A cup of cocoa contains approximately 170mg of theobromine.

The association of obesity with inflammation is now well established.

Given the impact of cocoa as a super food, why dark chocolate, with very high amounts of cocoa solids, is often limited - in weight loss diets – to a couple of squares is beyond me.

It can be eaten in greater quantities and more often than is normally advised.

Caffeine is also a methylxanthine. It is the main methylxanthine of coffee where it has alerting effects.

Its impact on the adenosine receptors is the reason why this stimulant keeps us awake if we drink it near bedtime.

On a personal level, I have found that when my intake of dark chocolate goes up replacing desserts – although the calories or more or less equal – I always lose significant amounts of weight during that period. This may also be due to another of the methylxanthines considerable therapeutic effects- that of acting as a diuretic.

One of my acquaintances who had been dieting for some time expressed surprise that they had lost 3lb one week. When I asked why they were surprised the response was that they had been eating a lot of chocolate that week.

It did not surprise me though.

This diuretic effect also has the ability to reduce blood pressure.   It seems that the positive impact that chocolate - containing very high amounts of cocoa solids has - extends far beyond what we initially assumed we knew.

In addition, given chocolate's ability to open airways, we are more likely to want to exercise since we will suffer less breathlessness when doing so.

What does the chocolate diet look like then? Is it something that we can fit into our busy lives without too much thinking about?

The answer is yes. Chocolate is a superfood and deserves more of a place in our lives but I am not talking about milk chocolate or white chocolate. Milk chocolate contains very little of the methylxanthines while white chocolate contains none at all. When I refer to chocolate for the purposes of the chocolate diet referred to in this book I am referring to the dark chocolate containing at least 85% cocoa solids.

I will also be referring to cocoa. When I refer to cocoa most people think I mean drinking chocolate but drinking chocolate is not pure cocoa.

However, a word in favour of milk chocolate. This is still a low glycaemic food and does not raise insulin levels in the way that fruit does.

If ounce for ounce you ate chocolate and fruit, you would not feel hungry after eating the chocolate but would after eating the fruit.

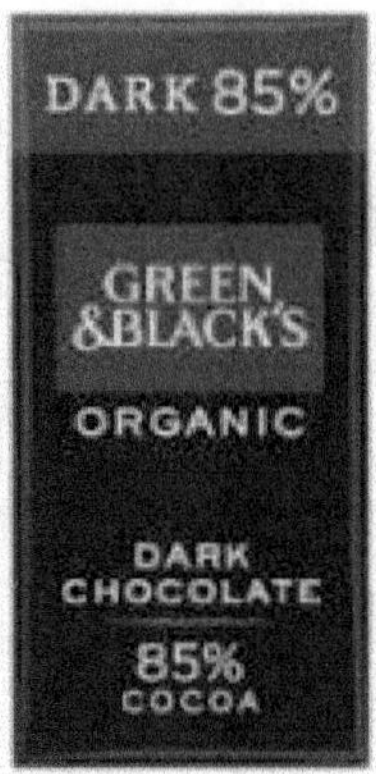

Most of drinking chocolate is sugar and cannot be used for dietary purposes at all.

 When I refer to cocoa I mean just that, pure cocoa solids without any added sugar. Pure cocoa can be a little bitter so sweetener may be added to taste at any time.

Now that we have established what our sources of methylxanthines are to be, it is quite likely you want to quickly discover how quickly – and well -the chocolate diet can fit into a daily regime. However, we need to look at some further amazing properties that the chocolate diet can bring.

 To this end we will look at chocolate as a polyphenol in our weight management programme. However, it may be useful to look at the diversity of nutrients that high quality chocolate contains.

In a 100g bar of chocolate there can be found

- 60% of the recommended daily intake (RDI) of iron (please note that iron cannot be absorbed without the addition of vitamin C).
- Over half of the RDI of magnesium
- 89% of copper (copper is an excellent antibacterial)
- Nearly the full RDI for manganese
- 11g of fibre (please note though that due to the high iron content of chocolate, it can be constipating)
- The fats are mostly saturated which means that they are stable and therefore do not cause inflammation.
- Chocolate also contains some beneficial monounsaturated fats, too.

In addition, there are many other nutrients in lesser quantities. High quality chocolate is really a superfood.

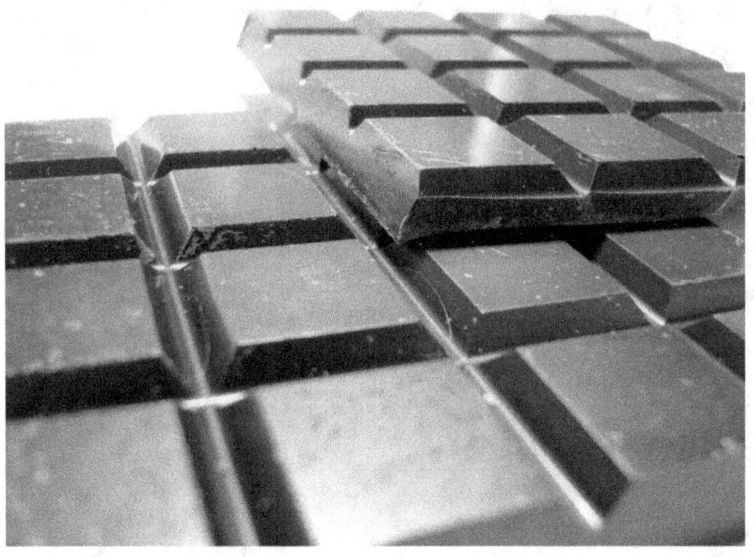

Dark chocolate really can be used in a weight reducing diet. One bar could even be used as a meal replacement.

Berberine and choline as weight reducing aids

Eating habits are notoriously difficult to alter. Benefits may be slow to appear and reduce motivation. It is easy to fall off the bandwagon. However, there are two supplements - choline and berberine- that address different aspects of metabolic syndrome. Together, they provide the perfect partnership for their ability to modulate all aspects of metabolic syndrome.

Berberine is a naturally occurring compound found in many plants such as goldenseal and the berberis shrub.

It is a popular over the counter medication in China where it is used for gastrointestinal infection.

It is a bitter tasting alkaloid yellow solid. For this reason, it is often taken in capsule form.

Studies, have shown that berberine works in a similar way to prescription drugs. Indeed, berberine has been found to be as effective as Metformin which is a well- known prescription medication used in diabetes treatment for lowering blood sugar levels.

Berberine travels to cells and activates an enzyme known as AMPK. AMPK controls many metabolic pathways.

These include those that help to inhibit the synthesis of cholesterol – including LDL cholesterol known as the bad cholesterol - and those which modulate insulin secreted by beta cells found in the pancreas.

Insulin resistance occurs as an impaired response to insulin.

 Insulin transports glucose to cells to be used for energy. However, resistance to insulin means that this function is limited. Blood sugar levels rise resulting in greater insulin production by the body in an attempt to overcome this.

Increased hunger, higher blood pressure and further weight gain are characteristic of insulin resistance.

Berberine helps address insulin resistance and rising blood sugar levels. However, it also aids the breakdown of sugar required for energy inside cells and the liver. This provides a readily available supply of energy for the body to use.

Triglycerides, the main component of body fat, also decrease after berberine supplementation.

A study of 37 obese men and women with metabolic syndrome found that 300mg of berberine given three times daily resulted in a BMI reduction from 31.5 to 27.4 within 3 months.

 This meant that the participants dropped from the obese to the overweight category.

 Part of this reduction in body fat was found to be due to an increase in leptin levels.

 Leptin is a hormone which has an appetite suppressing effect.

Berberine's ability to impact many pathways, involved in the manifestation of metabolic syndrome, means that weight reduction is achieved more easily.

The recommended dose of berberine is 500mg taken three times daily half an hour before meals.

Supplementation with berberine may induce mild gastrointestinal discomfort but this tends to be short-lived.

Choline is a recently discovered substance. It is an essential nutrient and although some in made in the body, most of it will need to be obtained from food.

Deficiency is common.   Although not a vitamin, choline has a number of characteristics in common with vitamin B complex.

Choline aids weight loss on a number of levels. Choline is needed for phosphatidylcholine synthesis which is a substance that prevents accumulation of fats in the liver.

Choline helps the body to use fat as a fuel by bringing fats out of the liver to be used for energy. Further, it helps to remove excess fat from the blood.

When fat is used as a fuel then hunger does not occur.

Studies on the effect of choline supplementation on rapid weight loss in female taekwondo and judo athletes have borne its weight reducing effects out.

Many athletes need to lose weight before important matches.

This study investigating the impact of choline on weight reduction was undertaken using a number of nutritional substances including choline.

The athletes took 2 doses of 1g of choline daily for one week. The results indicated a 10.23% change in loss of body fat. The results supported the hypothesis that choline could be used to lose weight rapidly without the loss of muscle mass which often occurs during calorie reducing diets.

Other studies have shown that supplementing with choline actually increases muscle mass while a deficiency has been found to cause muscle damage.

Retention or increasing muscle mass is important for weight loss as muscle tissue burns two and a half times more calories, when at rest, than fat does.

Studies have also shown that choline decreases plasma glucose level and the need for insulin which aids fat storage.

Good sources of choline are eggs and liver. A Recommended Daily Allowance has not been established for choline since it is a newly discovered substance. However, an Adequate Intake has been accepted. This is:

- 425mg for women
- 550mg for men

Two eggs provide about half of the choline requirements for the day.

Individuals who are at risk of choline deficiency include:

- Those with poor diets
- Those with malabsorption problems such as individuals with Crohn's disease
- Pregnant and nursing mothers
- The elderly

- Vegetarians and vegans

Berberine and choline exert their effect through different metabolic pathways. Between them they address the cornerstones of metabolic syndrome by reducing blood fats, cholesterol, insulin resistance and weight.

Their combined effect, in addition to healthy eating, is greater than the sum of their separate parts.

Their ability to collectively suppress hunger and supply a ready source of energy can make dieting appear effortless eliminating the 'hunger headache' and listlessness that often accompanies a calorie restricted diet and which is counterproductive.

Most of the time restricting adenosine and supplementing with choline and berberine takes care of most dietary needs.

Sometimes, there may be insulin resistance and this will stop weight loss.

Insulin resistance occurs when the cells cannot use the glucose building up in the blood stream.

The body does not want too high levels of glucose in the bloodstream since it can damage organs such as the eyes and kidneys.

More insulin is produced in an attempt to lower blood sugar levels.

This has the effect of increasing hunger and storing fat.

A short fast of up to three days, can reset this resistant phase back to normal working.

One to three days of fasting is a small price to pay for a lifetime of health.

There are a number of types of fast. These include:

- The water only fast
- The green salad fast

Sometimes just fasting for 16 hours a day- and eating normally in the eight hours' window that is left - works very well for some people.

In the end it is trial and error because everyone has a different genetic make-up and what works for one person will not definitely work for the next.

Food cravings are another of those diet spoilers. They tend to hit at a time when you have done particularly well sticking to an eating plan.

My cousin described how he could easily eat a bag of Liquorice Allsorts. After that, he could get back on track for a couple more weeks before it happened again.

He still managed to lose weight on this peculiar see saw of a diet.

Actually, it is not so odd. Many people have these cravings. Sometimes, you can see they make sense like craving fruit when you are short of vitamin C.

Not everyone is an expert on nutrition though so trying to identify the missing nutritional substance is not easy for most people.

Here is a chart to help you

Table showing typical craving, nutrient required and alternative or source of that nutrient

craving	Nutrient needed	Sources of nutrient or alternative food
Chocolate (I am unlikely to	magnesium	Dark chocolate,

swap this but alternatives are given)		nuts, seeds, green leafy vegetables
Salty foods	Chloride silicon	Fatty fish and goats milk Nuts and seeds
Carbs such as bread and pasta	nitrogen	Nuts, fatty fish and meat
Oily foods	calcium	Dairy products, broccoli, green leafy vegetables
Sugary foods	• Chromium • Carbon • Tryptophan • Phosphorus	Broccoli, grapes, cheese and chicken Fresh fruit Cheese, raisins, spinach and sweet potatoes Chicken, beef, fatty fish, dairy, nuts and grains

	• sulphur	Brussels sprouts, onions, garlic, cauliflower

Palmitic acid – one to watch

Palmitic acid is the most common saturated fatty acid and accounts for a total 20-30% of the total fatty acids in the body.

Palmitic acid can be made within the body by *de novo* lipogenesis or it can be obtained from food.

If too much in food is eaten. then its biosynthesis is generally reduced. This maintains optimum levels in body tissues.

Palmitic acid may need to be in a specific ratio to omega 6 and omega 3 fatty acids to maintain membrane phospholipids.

However, if there are too many mono and disaccharide carbohydrates in the diet and little exercise studies have stated that the palmitic acid concentration may be disrupted resulting in:

- dyslipidemia
- hyperglycaemia
- increased ectopic fat accumulation
- increased inflammation

The conclusion of the study was that when there is an imbalance of palmitic acid to PUFA ratio then de novo lipogenesis can flourish.

Significant amounts of palmitic acid can be found in these products:

- palm oil and products that contain palm oil such as pastry, crackers, fried potatoes, chips etc
- milk and milk products such as butter, cream, ice cream, sour cream, yoghurt, cheese and so on
- red meat and poultry
- coconut and coconut oil
- egg and egg products
- nuts
- avocado
- wheat and wheat products
- cocoa butter

Now we must not forget that some palmitic acid is vital for cell wall synthesis and it is the imbalance that causes problems.

The accepted intake of palmitic acid is 20-30g.

To give you an idea of the amount of palmitic acid there is in foods, I have included a small table with common foods in it.

Table showing foods and the percentage content of palmitic acid

Eggs (each)	22%
Cocoa butter	24-30%
Red meat	26%
chicken	22%
Full fat milk	21%

To work out how many grams of palmitic acid you have had

You find the weight of the product. For the purposes of this example we shall use a 170g prime beef burger.

26% of this beef burger is palmitic acid so we write the whole equation like this.

26/100 X 170g = 44.2g of palmitic acid

This is nearly twice as much as you require daily and it doesn't even take into account all the other food you are going to eat during the day.

The tissue content of palmitic acid influences *de novo* lipogenesis (DNL). Some nutritional factors, do too.

Disrupted homeostatic control of tissue concentration of palmitic acid can lead to:

- atherosclerosis
- neurodegeneration
- cancer

Carbohydrates eaten that are more than the capacity of the body to store as glycogen will stimulate lipogenesis. Therefore, eating fewer carbohydrates does really aid weight loss

Beware of Fruit

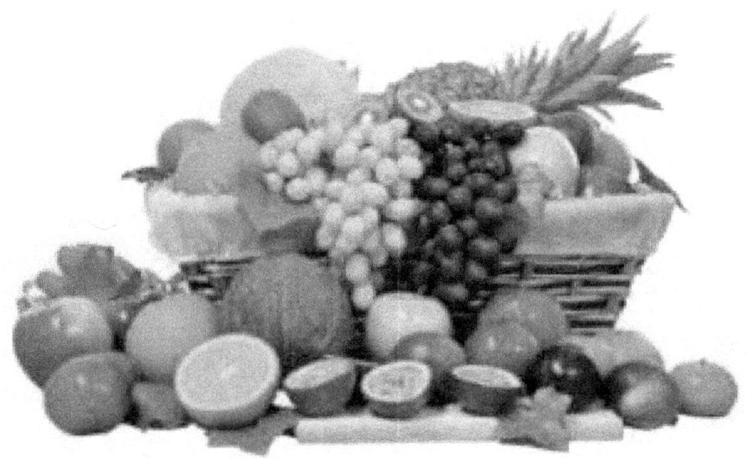

Now most people have been indoctrinated into the idea that fruit is great and the more fruit that you eat the better.

Now is the time to dispel that myth.

I understand that fruit has great antioxidants and we need to eat a variety of colours and that may be good for people who are skinny as a beanpole but.......

Fructose –fruit sugar- is taken up by the liver and cannot be used for biosynthesis.   As such it is promptly converted to a substrate used for making new fat cells.

It also likely contributes to non-alcoholic fatty liver disease.

High fructose foods include:

- apples
- grapes
- watermelon
- asparagus
- zucchini
- peas

Lower fructose foods are:

- bananas
- blueberries
- strawberries
- carrots
- green beans
- lettuce

There are also many foods that contain hidden sources of fructose.

You need to start label watching. If the product you wish to buy contains:

- molasses
- palm or coconut sugar
- fructose
- high fructose corn syrup
- agave syrup
- honey
- invert sugar
- sorghum[5]
- maple syrup or maple-flavoured syrup

then you need to find a substitute.

The flapjack that you buy from the supermarket may contain fructose but the one you make at home is unlikely to. Homemade is often best.

You might be surprised to find out how many common food stuffs contain high fructose corn syrup. It is a slow poison and will in the meantime make you look not one bit attractive.

Anyway, here is a list of the more common foods containing high fructose corn syrup.

- Sweetened yogurt
- Salad dressing
- Some brands of bread

---

[5] Sorghum is a plant with diverse uses including animal fodder and biofuel. It is also grown for its sugar content

- Canned fruit
- Granola bars
- Juice
- Junk foods like pizzas and ready meals
- Snack bars
- Cereal bars
- Nutrition bars

Now please do not think that I am saying do not ever have a granola bar again. I am not saying that at all.

Just find one that does not contain a form of fructose or better still make your own.

Fructose is a major contributor to metabolic syndrome and should be avoided at all costs. It is quite possible to lose weight eating - weight for weight - the same food only one is sweetened with glucose and the other fructose.

There are plenty of fructose tables to be found on the internet but the one below is more than adequate.

All you need to do now is copy the list that is fructose by its various names. This you take to the shop so that you can shop intelligently.

Fructose Malabsorption
Sugar Chart

AVOID!!!	OK	Maybe?
Agave Syrup	Cane Sugar	Barley Malt Syrup
Aspartame	Confectioners Sugar	Beet Sugar
Brown Sugar	Dextrin	Brown Rice Syrup
Corn Starch	Dextrose	Date Sugar
Corn Sugar	Evaporated Cane Sugar	Maple Syrup
Corn Syrup	Glucose	Raffinose
Corn Syrup Solids	Raw Sugar	Sucrose
Fructose	Stevia	Xylitol
Fruit Juice Sweeteners	Table Sugar (if not beet	
High Fructose Corn Syrup	sugar)	
Honey		
Inverted Sugar		
Isoglucose		
Isomalt		
Levulose		
Malitol		
Molasses		
Molasses Sugar		
Saccharin		
Sorbitol		
Splenda		
Sucralose		
Sucrose Syrups		

By now, you are probably thinking that you have far too much information. Should you tackle your fructose intake or eat more chocolate or……..

I would always seek to eliminate as much fructose as possible but I would start on that hidden in foods like mayonnaise and flapjacks; things like that.

Eating chocolate and reducing fructose are not mutually exclusive. It is quite possible to decide that you can only

---

[6] https://www.pinterest.co.uk/pin/421086633881510057/

manage to change two factors in your diet and just go for those.

Eventually, they will become second nature and you may want to add another change to your new eating pattern.

It can be seen that obesity is not just a matter of overeating. Not all calories are equal as we have been repeatedly informed over the years.

The source of the calories may increase blood sugar levels or promote lipogenesis and others may not.

This is probably why some people remain thin even though they appear to eat lots and others who appear to eat very little, gain weight.

We ought to turn at this point to mood disorders that are able to increase the potential for over eating and the reasons why this should happen.

 This is a very common problem and we should not underestimate its impact on attempts to lose weight.

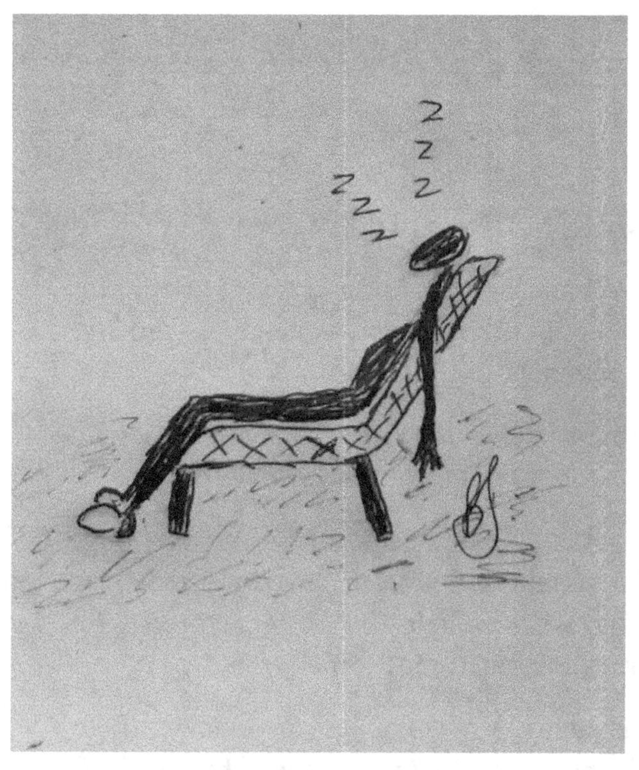

Eating too many carbohydrates will make you sleepy

Anxiety, stress and depression

All the above can increase appetite especially for carbohydrates that get broken down and converted into ready sources of energy.

This is a response to perceived threat. We eat in case we need energy to either fight an enemy or flee from them.

Our environment is still full of threats but not the ones that we physically fight or flee from. We do not use that extra energy that we have ingested. It gets stored to be used when a real physical threat comes along.

Of course, that does not make us less anxious but there are better responses that do not cause weight gain.

If we sprinkle gelatine on our food or stir a teaspoon into a drink, then this will have a calming effect.

Drinking tea also helps soothe – as if we didn't know this – as it contains a substance known as theanine which has a calming effect.

Tryptophan, the precursor of the feel good hormone, can be found in beans and lentils so when anxiety – or sleeplessness strikes, try a mug of lentil or bean soup.

Keeping a stock in the freezer is a good move.

Our friend, magnesium, also has a calming influence so eating foods that contain a lot of magnesium will also help avoid bingeing.

Lentil soup recipe – for calming thoughts

Take one cupful of red lentils

add to chopped onion, garlic, celery and chopped potato which has been fried for five minutes

fry for a further one minute

add seasoning and two cups of chicken stock

cook gently until the lentils are cooked and creamy

whizz all up in the blender

Add a dollop of yogurt before serving

Tip: some lentils may need soaking before you can add them to the ingredients above. However, the red lentil is one that doesn't need soaking and, to my mind, makes the best soup.

You can always add a sprinkle of gelatine for extra comfort.

The glycine in gelatine and the tryptophan in lentils both use different pathways to produce their calming effect.

If I had a fractious baby, I would give them cooked lentils.
It worked at calming them down in minutes.

Low potassium and the pot belly

This chapter has been taken from the book Causes of Weight Gain in EDS by Lynne D M Noble

Potassium is an essential mineral that impacts many areas connected with weight gain. Potassium is required for:

- The regulation of fluid in your body
- Maintaining mineral balance in and out of cells
- The normal contraction of muscles
- Normal blood pressure
- The assembly of protein and muscle from amino acids
- The maintenance of the acid base balance
- The control of the electrical activity of the heart
- The breakdown and use of carbohydrates for energy

It is well recognised that the sodium in salt causes fluid retention and the more potassium that is consumed the more fluid is excreted.

Numerous studies have shown that weight loss is higher in those with higher intakes of potassium. In addition, there is a trend for lower prevalence of metabolic syndrome and obesity with a higher consumption of potassium in the diet.

Potassium doesn't just help with weight loss though through this avenue. Potassium helps build bigger muscle. Greater muscle mass burns more calories.

Potassium also boosts metabolism and energy, burning more calories in the process.

Diuretics and potassium deficiency

It is not just those whose diets lack potassium that are at risk of weight gain. Individuals who use thiazide diuretics are also at risk of potassium deficiency. Thiazide diuretics such as Indapomide decrease serum potassium and glucose metabolism with an increased risk of diabetes and this risk tends to worsen with age.

The weight gain comes about because the glucose intolerance occurs as response to reduced insulin release and peripheral insulin resistance.

When insulin secretion is impaired the Beta cells, that produce insulin, aren't so responsive to glucose. The end result of this is abdominal obesity.

Many of the symptoms of impaired glucose tolerance go unnoticed. They may be put down to the effects of the diuretic tablets if they are recognised but individuals generally do not realise the significance of these.

Signs of impaired glucose tolerance include:

- Thirst
- Urinary frequency
- Dry mouth
- Tiredness/drowsiness
- Loss of muscle mass
- Blurred vision

Potassium supplements are never recommended. They are only allowed to be sold in very small doses and it is far easier to obtain potassium from food if you know which food contain them.

Tomatoes, tomato juice and paste are excellent sources of potassium as are bananas.

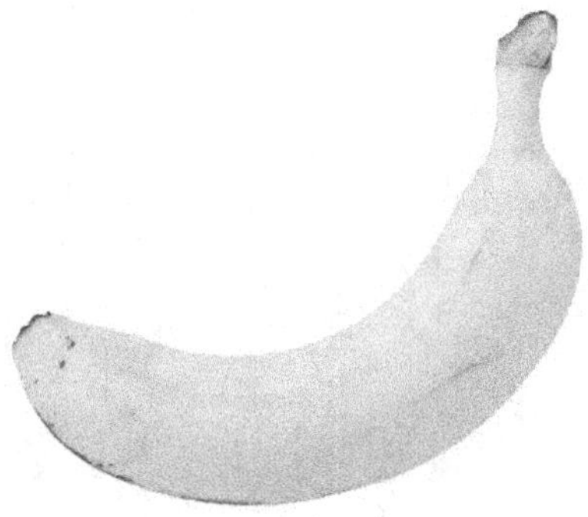

Bananas are a good source of potassium

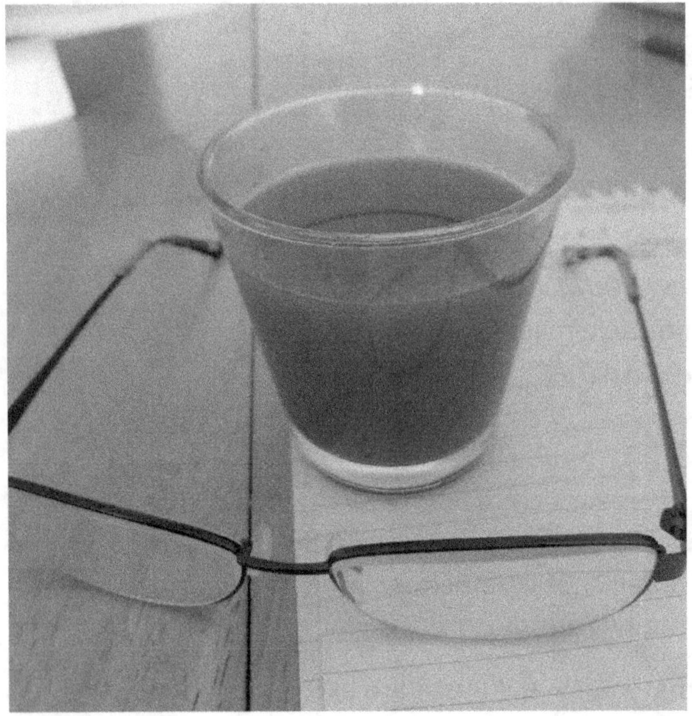

 Tomatoes in any form are an excellent source of potassium, too

The recommended daily allowance, of potassium for adults is:

Men: 4300mg

Women 3500 mg

Older adults may require slightly less as the kidneys find potassium harder to remove as you age.

Good sources of potassium apart from tomato products are:

- Dark green leafy vegetables such as spinach and chard
- Bananas
- Most fruits
- Broccoli and Brussels sprouts
- Pulses
- Nuts and seeds
- Meats – poultry and beef

Now, as I mentioned at the beginning of this book, my cousin has metabolic syndrome and diabetes.

Diabetes and metabolic syndrome is reversible with a little help and encouragement regarding diet. However, my cousin was put on increasing numbers of medications.

These are common medications for conditions associated with metabolic syndrome and diabetes. They can often worsen the condition that they are being taken for.

There can be some pretty nasty side effects too.

It might be worth looking at these medications.

The Medications

These are common medications used in conditions associated with metabolic syndrome.

- **Simvastatin**
- **Doxazosin**
- **Indapomide**
- **Amlodipine**
- **Irbersartin**

Some of their side effects are quite shocking.

Simvastatin

Simvastatin is a commonly used statin used for lowering the supposedly bad cholesterol known as LDL.

Cholesterol is a waxy substance which our bodies make naturally. It is made in the liver and is made in far greater quantities than we ever take in through diet. If we were to eat a high cholesterol meal our liver would just make less to restore the status quo. Cholesterol is an essential molecule without which there would be no life; virtually every cell in the body is capable of synthesising it.

Cholesterol is a major structural molecule which other major structural molecules are made from; as such it is a component in:

- o Bile acids which help to emulsify fats before digestion
- o Helps to make vitamin D which has hundreds of roles to play in the human body including bone building
- o synthesising an antimicrobial called cathelicidin and regulating the immune system thereby reducing the chances of an auto immune disease.
- o Steroid hormones (including sex hormones) are all cholesterol based.
- o It forms part of the myelin sheath that surrounds nerves and helps to carry messages.
- o Other steroid hormones produced from cholesterol include cortisol. This hormone helps to regulate blood sugar levels and defending the body against infection. Aldosterone, another hormone produced from cholesterol, helps retain salt and water in the body.
- o Cholesterol is required for forming memories. The information leaflets that accompany statins state that one of the side effects of statins is memory loss.

o Studies have shown that cholesterol neutralises toxins produced by bacteria. This may be why it is found at the site of arterial injuries. Of course some pathogens are able to cross the blood brain barrier, invade the brain, instigate neuro-inflammation and consequently neurodegeneration. Other pathogens which normally do not cross the blood brain barrier may if the brain is injured in some way. This is what we are wanting to avoid in the first place. Cholesterol helps protect and repair the brain.

We shall look at some of the above in more detail later. Meanwhile it is probably better to dispel the myth of 'good' and 'bad' cholesterol. The LDL and HDL that most people are familiar with are actually lipoproteins – not cholesterol. That is, they are made from a combination of a fatty molecule (not cholesterol) and a protein molecule. Lipoproteins are like rafts carrying cholesterol to where it is needed (low density lipoprotein) or taking away any excess (high density lipoprotein raft) when it is not needed.

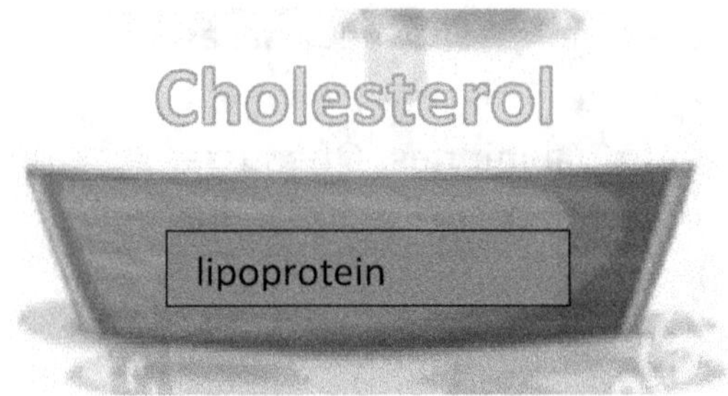

Medics do not like LDL scores to be higher than HDL scores. However, there are numerous studies showing that high LDL is correlated with better memory and increased longevity.

A recent study found that better memory and thinking was found in the over 85's in spite of high cholesterol.[7]

This has been replicated in other studies numerous times over.

In fact, it is the cholesterol carried on LDL – not HDL - that is linked with better cognitive function as you age. Why, in that case would you want to lower your LDL?

---

[7] https://www.alzheimersresearchuk.org/better-memory-thinking-seen-85s-despite-high-cholesterol/

The best marker for the small dense LDL that is associated with atherosclerotic plaque is the C-reactive protein test, not the one that tests cholesterol scores. They don't distinguish between the beneficial and harmful types of LDL.

C-reactive protein is a marker for inflammation. It is a strong indicator of future cardiovascular and neurological events.

High C-reactive protein can also be found during

- During times of high blood sugar levels
- Infection
- Obesity
- When blood is sticky (generally associated with high homocysteine (Hcy) levels.

I shall look at homocysteine, a little later among other substances that stimulate inflammation.

Did the well-respected Framingham Mass study reveal any alarming findings about cholesterol or saturated fat then?

William Castelli M.D. wrote this which appeared in the Archives of Internal medicine.

In Framingham Mass, the more saturated fat one ate, the more cholesterol one ate, the more calories one ate,

the lower the person's serum cholesterol .... we found that people who ate the most cholesterol, ate the most saturated fat [and] ate the most calories, weighed the least and were the most physically active.

In spite of a robust trail of research that showed that cholesterol was vital for human health and optimal levels had been artificially lowered, manufactures jumped on the bandwagon and started producing plant based health drinks and margarines that promised to lower cholesterol levels.

These, of course, came at a price.

The soluble fibre found in oatmeal, many fruits and lentils, for example, is applauded as being able to reduce levels of cholesterol. It can do this because it is not absorbed in the intestine and so binds to cholesterol and removes it from the body.

Once manufacturers realised that their products could reduce cholesterol, the prices of their goods went up.

Lowering cholesterol levels, through the use of statins, has not been proven to have prevented even one heart attack, studies have shown.

High cholesterol levels are associated with increased longevity and impact positively on the structure and function of the brain. Cholesterol, for example, has a critical role to play in the transmission of neurotransmitters. This means they pass messages on.

 Acetylcholine, for example, is necessary for motor control, learning, memory, sleep and dreaming.

Low levels of acetylcholine have been found in those diagnosed with Alzheimer's disease.

 Statins have been associated with an increase in motor neuron disease. Indeed, the sharp rise in ALS, the most common form of motor neuron disease which occurred in the 1990's, also coincided with the time when statins were heavily marketed.

One of the points I should make right at the start is that LDL has some beneficial properties especially for older people. For example, memory and cognition is better if you have elevated LDL.

Your immune system functions better because cholesterol is required to synthesise immune system cells involved in dealing with infection.

If your cholesterol levels are too low. then you are more likely to get – and die from - gastrointestinal and respiratory infections.

Statins can also cause long standing depression.

It is simply madness to mess about with perfectly good substances when the cholesterol score is a couple of points above what is an arbitrary reference range, anyway.

The upper limit for an acceptable cholesterol score happens to be five. However, studies have shown that a score of seven is the optimum level – in women anyway.

When you examine the benefits of cholesterol and the damage that statins can do, then the necessity of taking it is called into question.

Doxazosin

Doxazosin is a medicine prescribed to treat symptoms of an enlarged prostate and also high blood pressure. However, the latter is not its primary function.

It is what is commonly known as an alpha blocker.

Alpha blockers work to lower blood pressure by keeping the hormone norepinephrine from tightening the muscles in the walls of smaller arteries and veins.

It reduces blood pressure by relaxing blood vessel walls so that blood can pass through more easily.

This medicine is generally long term and this is usually for life.

There are many cautions in taking this medicine especially in the elderly.

Elderly people are classed as those aged over fifty-five years.

Side-effects[8]

Common or very common

Arrhythmias; asthenia; chest pain; cough; cystitis; dizziness; drowsiness; dry mouth; dyspnoea; gastrointestinal discomfort; headache; hypotension; increased risk of infection; influenza like illness; muscle complaints; nausea; **oedema**; pain; palpitations; skin reactions; urinary disorders; vertigo

Uncommon

Angina pectoris; anxiety; appetite abnormal; arthralgia; constipation; depression; diarrhoea; gastrointestinal disorders; gout; haemorrhage; insomnia; myocardial infarction; sensation abnormal; sexual dysfunction; stroke; syncope; tinnitus; tremor; vomiting; **weight increased**

How come most medications cause weight gain?

---

[8] https://bnf.nice.org.uk/drug/doxazosin.html

You can see that this medication can cause more problems than the problem it was originally prescribed for.

A diet with adequate potassium and magnesium normally sorts out any high blood pressure problems.

Indapomide

Indapomide is a diuretic. This means that it increases urination thereby reducing fluid in the blood vessels and body tissue.

In the process it helps eliminate potassium, magnesium and sodium along with excess fluid.

The fluid will then build up again but your body will be depleted of potassium and sodium and magnesium.

Since you need magnesium and potassium to lower blood pressure then this seems to be a pointless and dangerous exercise.

Side effects

The main side effects are the exacerbation of diabetes. When diabetes and metabolic syndrome (which is pre-diabetes) are the conditions we are trying to prevent, why is a medication given that worsens these conditions?

Adequate potassium intake and dark chocolate are very good diuretics.

- **Amlodipine**

Amlodipine is a calcium channel blocker (calcium antagonist) it works by relaxing and widening blood vessels by inhibiting the influx of calcium ions across the vascular smooth muscle and cardiac muscle.

Apart from magnesium and potassium though there are other foods that widen blood vessels and without the numerous negative side effects of this medication.

These include:

- Beetroot- a very good food to promote nitric acid synthesis
- Cocoa – this and chocolate are very good foods for promoting nitric acid synthesis
- Dark chocolate
- Leafy greens like kale, spinach and cabbage – the darker the better
- Organ meats
- Garlic

Two supplements that also widen blood vessels are coenzyme Q10 and L-arginine.

Coenzyme Q10 will almost certainly be deficient in those over the age of 55 years.

In addition, those taking statins will be undoubtedly deficient since statins prevent the synthesis of this enzyme.

L-arginine is an amino acid that is found in most sources of protein both animal and vegetable sources. However, the best food for L-arginine is turkey breast?

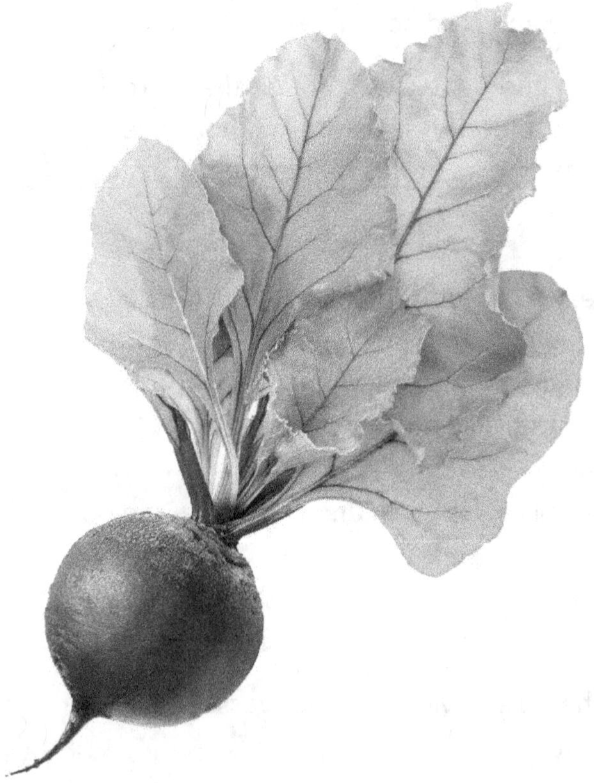

Beetroot is great for reducing blood pressure

The most common side effects include:

- headache
- flushing
- feeling tired
- swollen ankles.

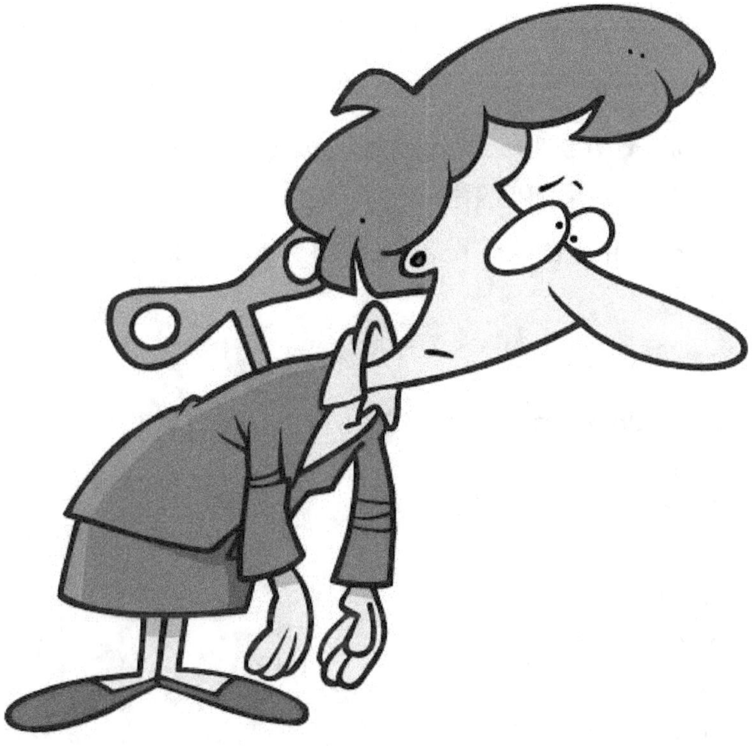

9

Amlodipine can make you feel very tired

---

9 http://clipart-library.com/tired-cliparts.html

Irbesartan

This medication is used to treat high blood pressure. It also helps to protect the kidneys from damage due to diabetes.

It belongs to a class of drugs called angiotensin receptor blockers also known as ARB's.

Angiotensin is a chemical that narrows blood vessels.

Blocking means that blood vessels widen and lower blood pressure in the process.

It helps prevent strokes, heart attacks and kidney problems.

Side effects include

- Musculoskeletal pain
- Chest pain
- Dyspepsia
- Flushing
- Hepatic disorders
- Sexual dysfunction
- Tachycardia
- Hypersensitivity
- Vasculitis
- Muscle cramps
- Taste altered
- tinnitus

There are many different metabolic pathways responsible for blood pressure regulation by means of Angiotensin Converting Enzymes (ACE). They are related to the following systems

1. Renin-angiotensin (RAS) also known as the renin-angiotensin-aldosterone system
2. Renin-chymase (RCS)
3. Kinin-nitric oxide (KNOS)
4. Neutral endopeptide (NEPS)

There are many food originating ACE inhibitors which include antihypertensive peptides.

Ace inhibitors derived from food proteins are the best known group of bioactive peptides

Dairy foods are excellent ACE Inhibitors.

They treat primary hypertension very well indeed.

Primary hypertension occurs due to life style factors like obesity and lack of exercise.

Secondary hypertension occurs due other medical conditions like kidney disease.

Now a little bit of chemistry here:

These antihypertensive peptides differ slightly at each end.

At one end is attached an amine group and this is called the N-terminal.

The amino acid residue on the other end has a carboxylic acid group attached to it and this is referred to as the C-terminal

Thus for simplicity

N------ | peptide | ———— **C**

There are specific amino acids residues which are typical for the N or C end of a peptide

The hydrophobic amino acids are characteristic of the N- end of a peptide and are specifically:

- Glycine
- Isoleucine
- Leucine
- valine

At the C end they are normally amino acids that are cyclic or have aromatic rings.

They comprise:

- proline
- tyrosine
- tryptophan

We can make good use of this knowledge for it now means that foods containing the above amino acids inhibit ACE thus preventing a rise in blood pressure.

It might be better to tabulate the different amino acids and look at good sources in food.

Table showing N terminal amino acids and their food sources

Amino acid residue	Food sources
Isoleucine	Beef chicken pork fish dairy beans lentil legumes whole grains seeds cocoa dark chocolate
Leucine	Chicken beef pork fish tofu canned beans milk cheese squash seeds and eggs
valine	beef chicken pork fish tofu yogurt beans podded peas seeds nuts and whole grains
glycine	any gelatinous compounds like gelatine, bone broth, organ meats

	meat with the skin or crackling left on

Table showing C terminal amino acids and their food sources

Amino acid residue	Food sources
Proline	Gelatin, chicken skin pork crackling proline milk soy protein
Tyrosine	Beef pork fish chicken tofu milk cheese beans seeds nuts and whole grains bananas
Tryptophan	Nuts seeds tofu cheese red meat chicken turkey fish oats beans lentil and eggs bananas

You will see that some of these foods are ones we have been told to avoid because they are bad for us such as pork crackling.

For further foods that contain these amino acids follow this link

https://nutritiondata.self.com/foods-000095000000000000000-w.html

These foods all contain ACE inhibitors and should be eaten on a daily basis when following the metabolic syndrome diet.

For chocolate lovers who are feeling left out, chocolate also contains the amino acid phenylalanine. This has an association with tyrosine – one of our C-terminal amino acid residues.

Phenylalanine is involved in making dopamine which is a brain chemical than can regulate mood.

It helps to stimulate the metabolism firing up the processes that give life

You will note that the tables do not include simple carbohydrates purely because simple carbohydrates do not contain the amino acids that we require to inhibit ACE that narrows blood vessels.

At the end of this long passage on foods that can replace blood pressure medications, we have learned some chemistry.

This stands us in good stead in understanding some of the many complex processes that underlie the mechanisms involving high blood pressure.

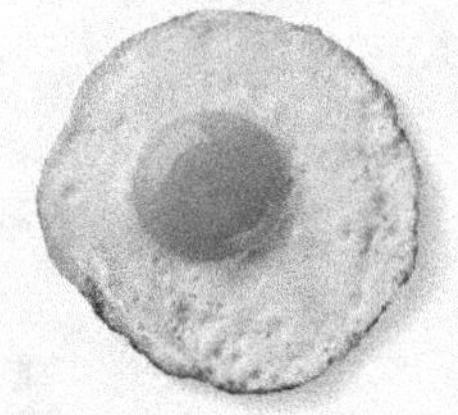

Eggs are a good source of N terminal amino acids

We come to our last medication.

Rivaroxaban

Rivaroxaban is a blood thinner or anticoagulant

It is taken if people have coronary heart disease or peripheral arterial disease among others.

Both of these conditions are associated with metabolic syndrome.

Side effects of this medication include:

- bleeding in the brain
- seizures
- changes to eyesight
- numbness or tingling
- tiredness, weakness
- feeling sick

there are a number of foods that are natural blood thinners and these include:

- turmeric
- ginger
- cinnamon (also lowers blood pressure)
- cayenne peppers
- vitamin E

WHOLE GRAINS

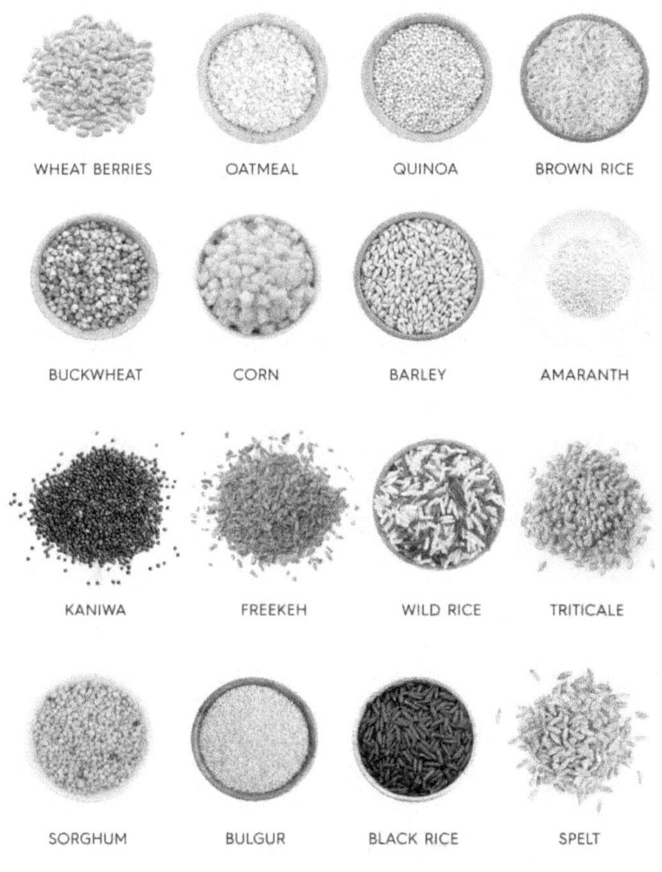

Vitamin E is found in nuts, wheat germ, nut oils and whole grain foods.

These can be eaten without the side effects that many prescribed medications bring with them.

What if I am already on prescribed medications?

If you already on prescribed medications, then clearly you cannot stop them overnight. You may get a rebound action so that your blood pressure temporarily jumps up if a medication is stopped.

Initially, you need to implement the diet that helps to reduce your body mass and blood pressure.

It is helpful if measurements for these and waist circumference are logged.

After a couple of weeks compare the measurements again.

They should all have improved.

Continue for another couple of weeks.

Compare your results

As your body mass and blood pressure reduces. Your medication could be reduced.

This is because when medication is first prescribed it is partly based on your symptoms and your body mass.

It may be that if your blood pressure was very high initially you may have been placed on an ACE and a diuretic.

One of these may now need to be withdrawn or at least a lower dose prescribed.

These reductions should be logged for they are great motivators when looking at the progress that has been made.

You will need to continue like this until you are not dependent on prescription medications to respond to conditions which are amenable to diet or, at the very least reduced them considerably.

Already, we have covered a lot of ground in looking how food can be our medicine.

Some people, like my cousin, will no doubt enjoy putting together recipes that address the many issues of metabolic syndrome that he has.

Others will struggle either because they do not have cooking skills, the will or motivation or the time.

This will then take a little more planning because the emphasis here is creating your own dishes from scratch.

The other difficulty that people may have is the concept that chocolate is bad and fruit is good for you.

I can only reiterate that chocolate is an excellent food and eating too much fruit can lead to weight gain.

When nutritionists have extolled the virtues of fruit it is generally in terms of antioxidants and the amount of vitamin C fruit may contain.

However, lightly cooked or raw vegetables contain plenty of vitamin C and little, if any, fructose so you can include asparagus, cauliflower, green peppers, broccoli, leafy greens, celery, mushrooms, white potatoes, shallots. Spinach. Peas, cucumber, beans and root vegetables in your diet.

Further, you may not realise that there are plenty of antioxidants in animal protein. They are not just the domain of fruits.

It might be useful to look at antioxidant minerals and vitamins

These are:

Vitamins – E, C and beta carotene

Minerals – copper, manganese, selenium and zinc

They all help to protect the body from free radicals which cause damage and inflammation in the body.

Selenium for example is used to make glutathione peroxidase which neutralises hydrogen peroxide in the body.

The best source of selenium is found in Brazil nuts.

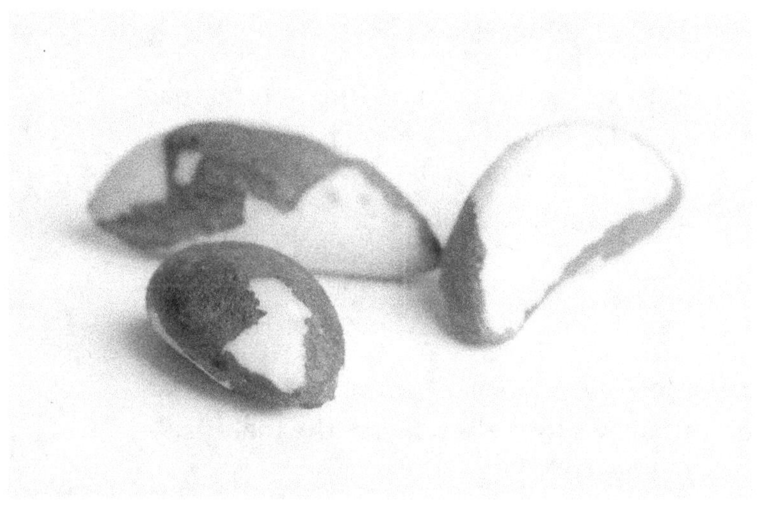

Two Brazil nuts provide all the recommended daily intake of selenium.

Autophagy

The value of autophagy as part of a treatment for disease conditions has been known for many years. Autophagy is a process in which old damaged cells are recycled in order to produce newer healthier ones.

Autophagy means 'self-eating.' In this process damaged cells are delivered to tiny organelles known as lysosomes.

Here the larger dysfunctional macromolecules are broken up. This allows the cells to reuse the materials in the synthesis of new cells.

Fasting has been shown to increase the generation of nerve cells as well as enhancing brain function.

The removal of old and dysfunctional proteins is a necessary process in cellular repair, across all types, including that of those found in the central nervous system.

Intermittent fasting has also been found to affect gene expression which results in changes to gene function. These changes are related to longevity as well as protection against disease.

Further benefits are to be found in insulin levels. Insulin levels improve and insulin drops rapidly. This drop in insulin levels make body fat more accessible to be burnt for energy.

Fasting increases HGH-X5. This substance aids fat loss and muscle gain.

Autophagy has a number of major implications for neurodegenerative disorders such as Alzheimer's Disease, motor neuron disease and multiple sclerosis. However, the effect of intermittent fasting on the build-up of amyloid beta protein – characteristic of Alzheimer's disease – is of particular interest.

Why should autophagy have the potential for such a beneficial effect?

One possible explanation is that the slow clearance of amyloid beta protein occurs in a high copper to zinc ratio.

Copper slows the removal of amyloid beta protein from the brain to the blood stream. It may be that intermittent fasting reduces the levels of copper in the brain.

Further, fasting drops insulin and increases glucagon which stimulates autophagy. This occurred after 14-16 hours of fasting. However, it is quite likely that other mechanisms are in play.

Given the many potential benefits of fasting, fasting for 14-16 hours twice weekly may be considered as a treatment for those with neurodegenerative disorders.

Vitamin D deficiency and weight gain

The role of vitamin D in human health has become studied more in recent years in relation to the inverse relationship between vitamin D levels and obesity.

These studies are important because approximately 80% of the world population are vitamin D deficient.

In one study 400 overweight and obese participants, with vitamin D deficiency were divided into three groups.

The first group did not receive vitamin D supplementation.

The second and third group received 25,000 and 100,000 IU's, monthly, respectively.

After 6 months it was found that the groups that had supplemented with vitamin D had lost weight and had smaller waists.

There are a number of reasons why this may have occurred.

In obesity, vitamin D increases insulin sensitivity and insulin sensitivity is associated with weight loss.

As vitamin D also affects the storage and production of fats, increasing vitamin D to restore levels back to optimum helps to decrease the body fat percentage.

Vitamin D also helps to address systemic inflammation.

Systemic inflammation is often associated with those who are obese with an apple shaped profile.

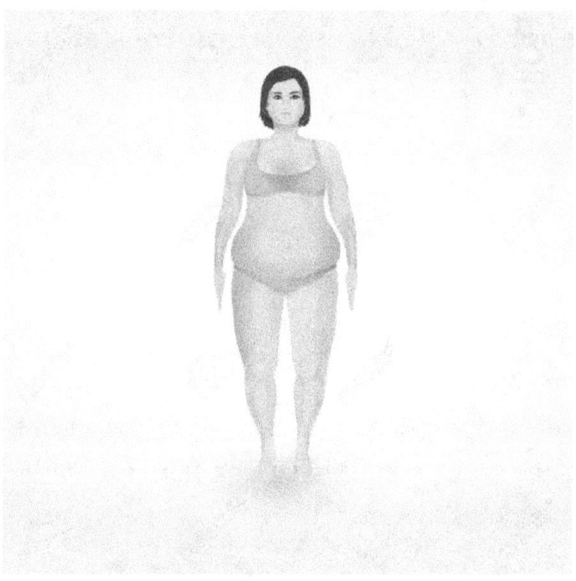

Typical apple shape [10]

---

[10] https://www.123rf.com/photo_53224488_stock-vector-apple-body-shape.html

Vitamin D activates receptors in the pancreatic beta cells. The main function of a beta cell is to produce and secrete insulin.

Insulin helps to regulate levels of glucose in the blood.

Vitamin D is practically impossible to get enough of in diet. There are so few sources. The main sources are:

- Oily fish
- Eggs
- Irradiated mushrooms
- Fortified cereals
- Lard

The sun provides the most vitamin D by its action on the skin but as we age, the mechanism by which this comes about is not as efficient. In addition, our ability to absorb nutrients also becomes less effective.

A number of groups of people are at particular risk of vitamin D deficiency. These include:

- The elderly (those over the age of 55 years)
- People of colour

- People with malabsorption problems such as those with Crohn's disease
- People who remain mainly indoors
- Those on low fat diets as vitamin D needs to be taken with a little fat in order for it to be absorbed.
- Those on a poor diet generally
- Obese people

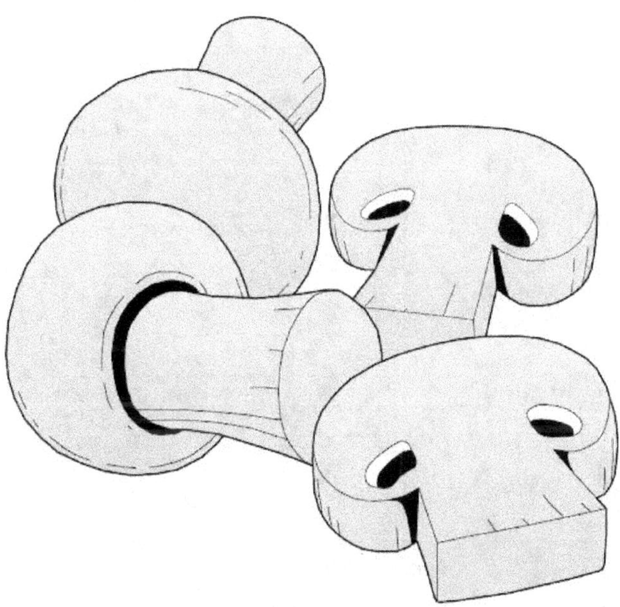

Irradiated mushrooms are a good source of vitamin D

Obese people are at risk because fat cells act as a storage reservoir for vitamin D. The more obese an individual is the greater the storage capacity when really we need vitamin D to be circulating in the body.

The signs of vitamin D deficiency include:

- Hair loss
- Osteopenia
- Osteoporosis
- Frequent infections
- Weight gain
- Fatigue
- Bone pain
- Depression
- Muscle cramps, weakness and aches
- Diabetes
- Autoimmune disease

The recommended daily allowance is 2,000 IU's. Vitamin D is a fat soluble vitamin and cannot be absorbed unless taken with a little fat.

One of the casualties of 'progress' is the discontinued use of lard which contains good amounts of vitamin D.

High blood pressure, chocolate, flavanols and the ACE 1 and 2 Receptors

We have already looked at some of the benefits of chocolate but, of course, this amazing food has even further benefits as it blocks the ACE1 doorway which makes highly inflammatory angiotensin II.

Firstly, it would be helpful to look at both ACE proteins – ACE I and ACE2 – and their functions. We will start off 'backwards' and look at ACE2 first.

The ACE2 is an enzyme that is attached to the cell membranes of the cells in many organs. These include:

- Arteries
- Intestines
- Lungs
- Heart
- kidney

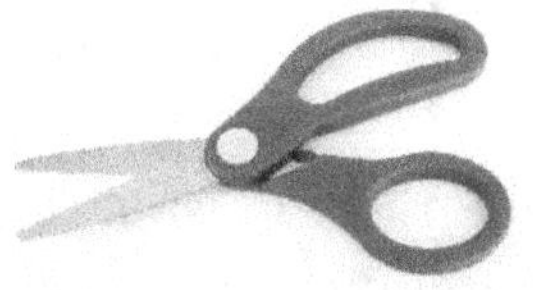

ACE2 helps cut up angiotensin II into smaller fragments

It helps cut up the larger protein angiotensin II into smaller molecules – angiotensin - which are used for other functions to counteract the effects of angiotensin II.

If angiotensin II was not reduced, then the knock on effect would be that blood pressure would increase. Further, the resulting inflammation would damage the delicate linings of the blood vessels and other tissue.

Therefore, ACE2 is an essential enzyme for regulating:

- blood pressure
- inflammation
- wound healing

It works through a pathway known as the renin-angiotensin-aldosterone system also known as the RAAS pathway.

However, some viruses block ACE2. They use ACE2 as a cellular doorway for entry into the host cell. When host cells become infected by virus then pro-inflammatory cytokines are expressed.

When this blocking occurs then the normal function of ACE2 cannot happen. The blood pressure increases and tissue damage occurs. When ACE2 receptors are blocked in the alveoli of the lungs, then massive tissue damage can occur.

The ACE1

In contrast, ACE1 promotes the formation of angiotensin II.

Both ACE enzymes normally work together to regulate blood pressure. In matters of high blood pressure this regulatory process does not always work.

Drugs called ACE inhibitors are sometimes prescribed. These impede the formation of angiotensin II.

Researchers have argued that it is the abnormally high production of angiotensin II that indicates the amount of damage that can be caused by certain viruses.

The good news is that these ACE1 receptors are significantly inhibited by a certain type of flavanol.

The even better news is that the main flavanols are found in cocoa and chocolate products as well as grapes,

Flavanols are a part of the class known as flavonoids.

Flavanoids are substances found in plants and fungi and their main functions are protective and include

- fight free radicals
- regulate the activity in your cell.

The flavonoids can be subdivided into flavonols and flavanols based on their structure. It is the latter flavanols that we are interested in.

These can be subdivided but the subgroup we are interested in include the catechins and epicatechins.

It is easier understanding the relationship through a diagram.

Diagram showing the flavonoids that help to lower blood pressure

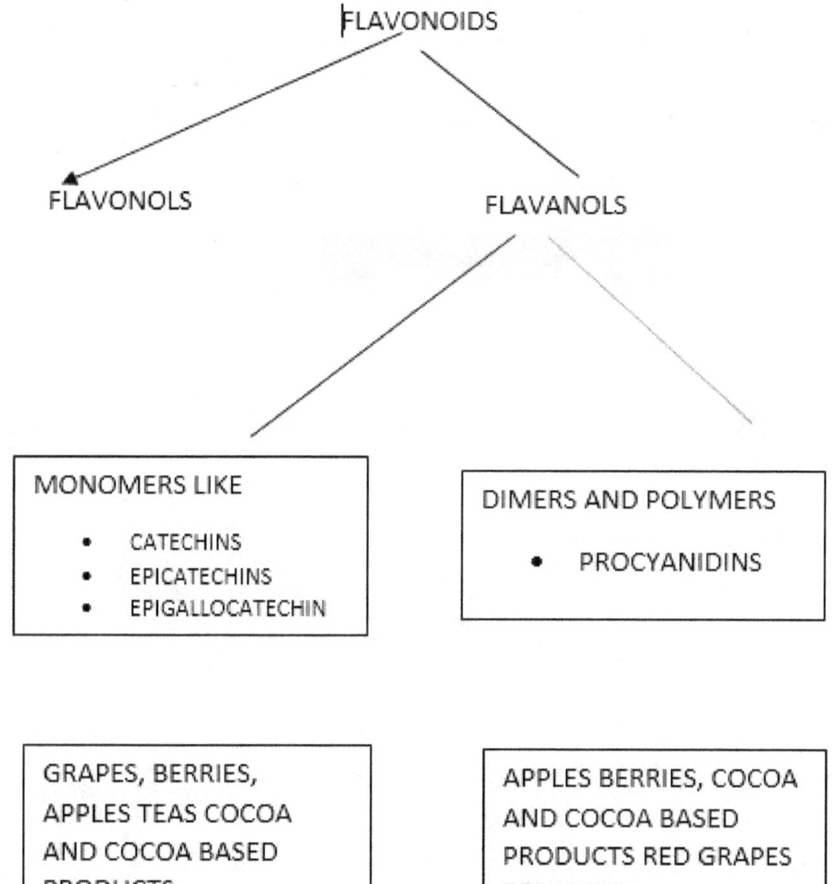

These glorious flavanols will help reduce blood pressure by inhibiting ACE1 from synthesising angiotensin II.

These flavanols come without the side effects that often come with prescribed medications and a diet rich in the above should, in my opinion, be tried first (along with foods containing potassium and magnesium) before resorting to prescription medicine.

Metabolic acidosis

Metabolic acidosis is implicated in many disease states yet very few people have heard of it or how it may impact health.

Metabolic acidosis develops when too much acid is produced in the body or if the kidneys and lungs are unable to remove enough acid from the body. The pH of the blood should be around 7.4 and anything lower is referred to as acidosis whilst anything higher is referred to as alkalosis.

Metabolic acidosis can cause serious health issues and may be life threatening.

The excess acid may occur due to lactic acid (produced during exercise) or ketoacids.

There are three main ways that ketoacidosis can come about. These are through:

- Alcohol
- Being in a diabetic state
- Starvation

I shall look at these in more detail later.

It may occur due to the loss of bicarbonate which may occur for a number of reasons including the ageing process.

It may occur due to the reduced ability of the kidneys and lungs to excrete excess acid. Therefore, people with lung conditions such as asthma or COPD, for example, are at particular risk.

As acidosis can start in the lungs or the kidneys then we can divide them into two separate categories. Each of them has their own specific symptoms and it is easier to compare them if they are tabulated for convenience.

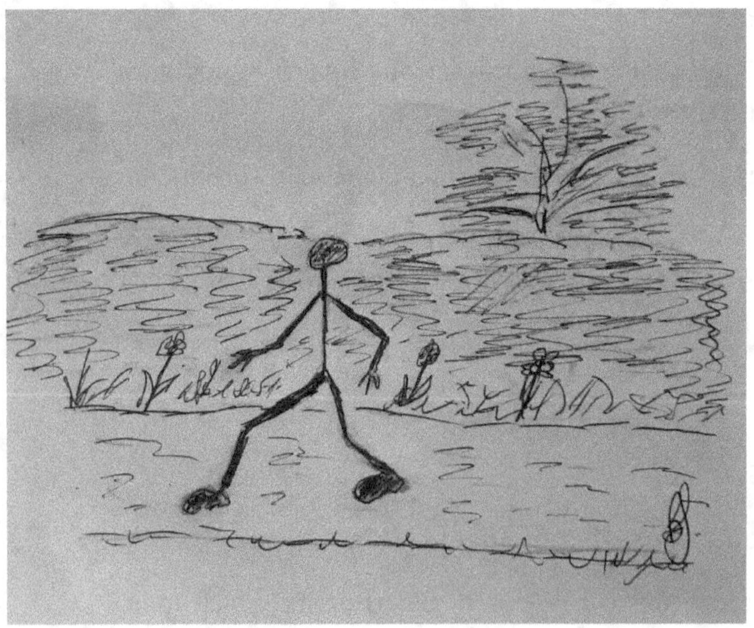

Excessive exercise can induce ketoacidosis

Table showing the symptoms of respiratory and metabolic acidosis

Respiratory acidosis	Metabolic acidosis
Drowsiness	fatigue
Easy fatigue	Confusion or severe anxiety due to hypoxia
Shortness of breath	Rapid shallow breathing
Headache	headache
sleepiness	Sleepiness coma lethargy decreased visual acuity
confusion	Loss of appetite nausea vomiting abdominal pain altered appetite weight gain
	Diabetic acidosis (breath smells fruity) and Kussmaul respirations (deep rapid breathing associated with diabetic ketoacidosis)
	jaundice
	Tachycardia (increased heart rate) abnormal heart rhythms (eg. ventricular tachycardia) and low blood pressure due to decreased response to epinephrine
	Joint and bone pain muscle weakness

I have already touched on the point that ketoacidosis can occur due to alcohol, a diabetic state and starvation. As diabetes - and the potential to starve oneself – is tied in with metabolic syndrome, then it would be wise to look at this condition a little further.

Diabetic ketoacidosis is a serious complication of diabetes. It develops when your body cannot produce enough insulin and ketones are produced as a source of energy from the breakdown of fat.

The signs of diabetic ketoacidosis are that blood sugar levels will be high (hyperglycaemia) as will ketones.

There are testing kits for both.

The symptoms of this condition include:

- More frequent urination
- Thirst
- Pear drop breath
- Drowsiness
- Stomach pain
- Feeling or being sick
- Confusion
- Passing out
- Deep fast breathing

Starvation ketosis occurs when the glycogen stores in the liver are exhausted and energy must be obtained from the breakdown of fat stores.

This may start between 15-24 hours of fasting or but gathers pace the longer the period of starvation.

Clearly, while we may want the weight loss, we do not want a state of acidosis with all the signs and symptoms that go with that.

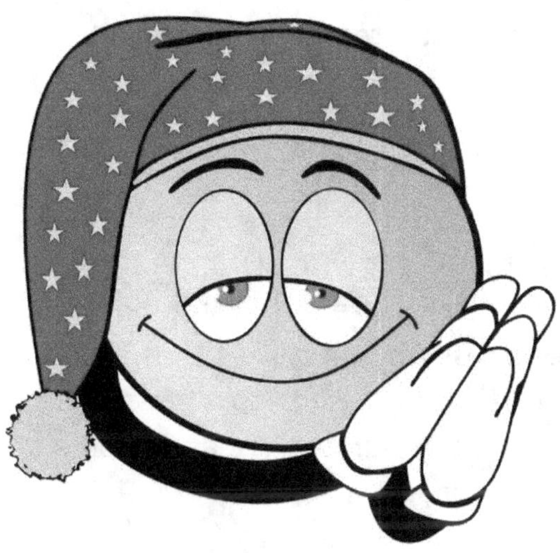

Metabolic acidosis can make you feel very sleepy

Dr Mark Sircus, in his book Sodium Bicarbonate Nature's Unique First Aid Remedy cites the dosage of sodium bicarbonate as provided by Arm and Hammer for oral use.

This is:

- Add half a teaspoon of bicarbonate of soda to half a glass of water and take every two hours

Do not take more than three half teaspoons if you are over 60 years of age.

Do not use this maximum dosage for more than two weeks.

As many of the problems that occur with dieting – such as headache and loss of energy – are due to the body being in a state of ketoacidosis then it makes sense to add one teaspoon of bicarbonate of soda to a glass of water and take this at any point during the day. If you prefer you can sip it over the day.

You may not lose huge amounts of noticeable weight during this time because the sodium can cause slight oedema. However, if you take plenty of foods containing potassium and magnesium this should counteract this tendency.

At the end of two weeks it is preferable if you reduce the sodium bicarbonate but there is always the option of increasing it if the symptoms of ketoacidosis occur.

The best way to test whether the body is in an acid state or not is through the use of saliva or urine tests.

To test for saliva, wait until 2 hours after eating then fill the mouth with saliva and test with litmus. It should go blue. A healthy alkaline state should be between 7.1 and 7.5.

Anything less than 7.1 places you   in an acidic state and needs to be remedied by the addition of some bicarbonate of soda in water as outlined above.

You can test as many times as you like for the pH.

With urine tests the expectation is that the pH range will be between 6.5 to 7.5 on the urinalysis strips. If the test reveals that the pH is lower, then you follow the regime mentioned above until a state of health returns.

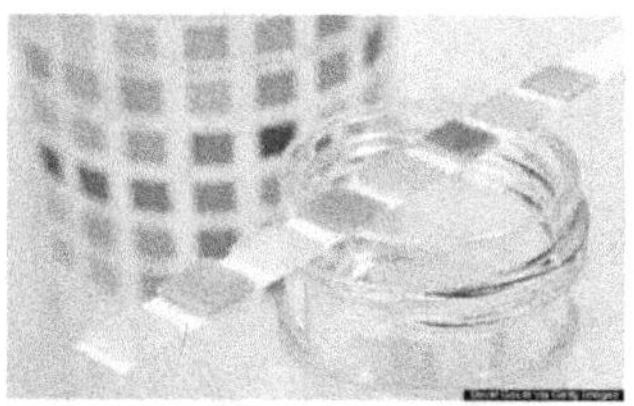

Urinalysis   is a straightforward process

All you need to do is dip the stick into fresh urine and read it off the chart you will find wrapped around the container.

Clearly, bicarbonate of soda is useful in preventing the lethargy and headachy type symptoms that often accompany the initial stages of a calorie controlled diet or diets which rely heavily on protein or fat and thus produce a state of acidosis.

However, there are no studies that have found that taking sodium bicarbonate will directly help with weight loss but as one of an arsenal of weapons it has considerable value.

 It is cheap, easily obtainable in any supermarket and it deserves a place in the overall strategic plan to recover from metabolic syndrome.

Its only drawback is that such simplicity may mean that it is overlooked as an adjunctive treatment for a complex condition that affects approximately one third of the population.

Final Thoughts

Losing weight is not all that the experts deem it to be.

Not all calories are equal, far from it. It very much depends on the source of those calories and whether they contain simple sugars that raise insulin levels or adenosine that prevents the breakdown of fat to be used for energy.

How we respond may be down to genetics.

We are taught that if we exercise then we will lose weight. This is not entirely true either if we are susceptible to the effects of adenosine which increases with exercise.

Walking is good for helping to stimulate lymph glands. It is good for cardiovascular health and building muscle mass – at least in the legs but you will not necessarily lose weight exercising.

We are taught to have a high protein breakfast as this is better for us but a 2012 Tel Aviv study in Israel found differently.

They put 200 volunteers on either a low carb meal or one that included carbs such as chocolate cake.

Both groups lost the same amount of weight but after another 4 months when there was more freedom over meal choices, the dessert eaters were still losing weight while the others were putting back on, the weight they had lost.

The reasoning behind this is because a dessert first thing in the morning is thought to lower levels of ghrelin which is the hunger hormone.

It also appears to reduce cravings for sugary foods later in the day.

Daniela Jakubowicz says that to get the best effect, the dieters should have a food they often crave for dessert at breakfast time.

If this is chocolate, then this is good news as serotonin levels are raised due to the tryptophan contained in the chocolate.

Serotonin, is of course, the feel good brain chemical.

I had also noticed well before this study came out that if I ate a bar of chocolate for breakfast then I was not in the least bothered about carbohydrates for the rest of the day.

This seemed to fly in the face of popular opinion at the time but it did cut down my intake of carbohydrates considerable throughout the day.

Of course, some people do feel better on their English breakfasts and that is what is right for them. We can never discount the influence of genetics.

But, in a similar vein we can never discount the influence that our cultural organisation has on our health.

We often sit down to eat three meals a day, regardless of whether we are hungry or not because that is what we have come to believe we **should** do.

I have bolded and italicised the word should because whenever we see that word it means that cultural expectations have crept into our thinking.

At this point, if we are wise, we might consider taking a step back and reflecting on why we do things and when.

Why do we think a croissant and jam is healthier than chocolate for breakfast when it clearly isn't on quite a number of counts?

The prescribed medications given to address metabolic syndrome can make the condition worse.

If the GP addresses one troubling symptom through medication. then ten negative side effects may be the result and worsen the whole outcome.

The diuretics build up visceral fat – the dangerous inflammatory abdominal obesity – by lowering potassium levels.

Low potassium levels can cause further heart problems, constipation, mood disorders and many other conditions that prevent life from being enjoyed to the full.

Food is a great medicine providing all the enzymes and macro and micro nutrients required to support life. It can positively impact your health far more than medications can ever do and without the concerning side effects that accompany over the counter and prescribed medicines.

I am grateful to my cousin for allowing me to use his story and for being so honest about the struggles. Without this knowledge I would not have been motivated to write this book which is of importance to one in four of people living in the UK.

I look forward to when he is not in a diabetic state and his blood pressure is not of concern. This is a reversible condition and he is improving week by week.

It is good to see.

An example of a daily record.

Date						
Weight						
Blood pressure						
Blood sugar						
Waist circumference						
Daily steps walked						
Wellbeing on a scale 1 to 10						
Notes						

Table 1[11]

Natural Compounds with Antihypertensive Qualities

Diuretics

- Vitamin B_6 (pyridoxine)

- Taurine

- Celery

- Gamma-linolenic acid

- Vitamin C (ascorbic acid)

- Potassium (K+)

- High gamma/delta tocopherols and tocotrienols

- Magnesium (Mg++)

- Calcium (Ca++)

---

[11] https://www.ncbi.nlm.nih.gov/pmc/articles/PMC3989080/

- Protein

- Fiber

- Coenzyme Q1 0

- L-carnitine

- Hawthorne berry

Calcium-Channel Blockers

- Alpha-lipoic acid

- Magnesium (Mg++)

- Vitamin B_6 (pyridoxine)

- Vitamin C

- Vitamin E: high gamma/delta E with alpha tocopherol, (high cytosolic Mg++ with low Ca++); also a diuretic

- N-acetyl cysteine

- Hawthorne berry

- Celery

- Omega-3 fatty acids (eicosapentaenoic acid and docosahexaenoic acid)

- Calcium

- Garlic

- Taurine

Beta Blockers

- Hawthorne berry

Angiotensin-Converting Enzyme Inhibitors

- Garlic

- Seaweed (wakame, etc.)

- Tuna protein/muscle

- Sardine protein/muscle

- Hawthorne berry

- Bonito fish (dried)

- Pycnogenol

- Casein

- Hydrolyzed whey protein

- Sour milk and milk peptides

- Gelatin

- Sake

- Omega-3 fatty acids

- Chicken egg yolks
- Zein
- Dried salted fish
- Fish sauce
- Zinc
- Melatonin
- Pomegranate

Central Alpha Agonists *(Reduced sympathetic nervous system activity)*

- Taurine

- Potassium (K+)

- Zinc

- Sodium (Na+) restriction

- Protein

- Fiber

- Vitamin C

- Vitamin B_6 (pyridoxine)

- Coenzyme Q10

- Celery

- Gamma-linolenic acid /dihomo-gamma-linolenic acid

- Garlic

Angiotensin-Receptor Blockers

- Potassium (K+)

- Taurine

- Resveratrol

- Fiber

- Garlic

- Vitamin C

- Vitamin B_6 (pyridoxine)

- Coenzyme Q10

- Celery

- Gamma linolenic acid/dihomo-gamma-linolenic acid

Direct Vasodilators

- Omega-3 fatty acids
- Monounsaturated fatty acids (Omega-9 fatty acids)
- Potassium (K+)
- Magnesium (Mg++)
- Calcium (Ca++)
- Soy
- Fiber
- Garlic
- Flavonoids
- Vitamin C
- Vitamin E
- Coenzyme Q10
- L-arginine
- Taurine
- Celery
- Alpha-lipoic acid

The Problem with Statins

(A more in depth look at a common medication generally prescribed to those with metabolic syndrome)

Statins were introduced into western medication in the late 1950's after concerns that high cholesterol may be linked with heart disease.

In spite of many robust studies that found that there wasn't a connection, healthy levels of cholesterol were artificially lowered thus medicalising a healthy state in an individual.

Cholesterol is synthesised in a metabolic pathway known as the Mevalonate Pathway (MP).

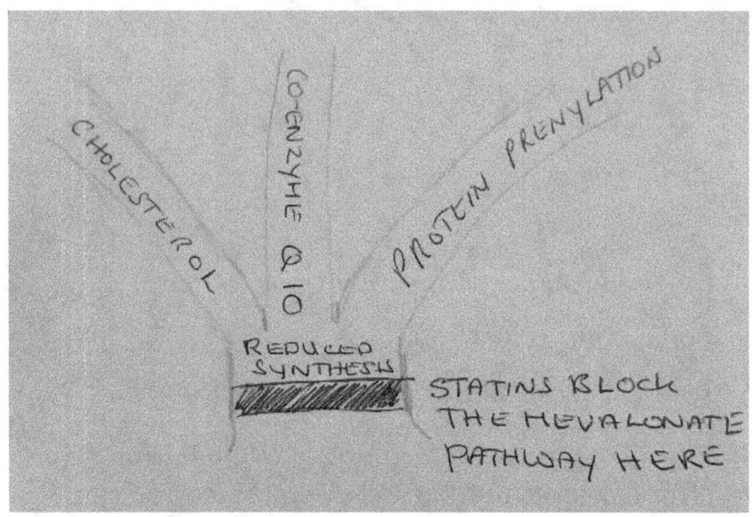

An enzyme known as HMG Co-A reductase is the role limiting enzyme of the Mevalonate Pathway

The MP is a huge branching network where many vital substances are made.

It makes essential constituents of cell as well as key metabolites.

Metabolites are small proteins that take part in chemical reactions. They are vital for changing food into energy which is used to enable us to grow, think, move, among other actions.

 Two other substances made in the MP, besides cholesterol, will be looked at later.

Statins block the MP at its root. As such, not only is the synthesis of cholesterol blocked but two other substances which for vital for health are disrupted.

These are:

Coenzyme Q10 and protein prenylation.

Protein prenylation is a process. It helps to localise certain proteins to membranes. If this process is disrupted it is associated with defective autophagy.

Autophagy is the process of cleaning up dead and damaged mitochondria. When this is incomplete it results in inflammatory activity and cell death.

Mitochondria are tiny cell organelles. They generate most of the energy that a cell needs to power its chemical reactions.

The disruption of protein prenylation is a significant risk factor for neurodegenerative disorders such as Alzheimer's disease. Therefore, the negative impact of statins, in this respect, is wide reaching.

Coenzyme Q10 (Q10) is an antioxidant which is used by cells for growth and maintenance. It is also necessary for a process known as bio-energetics.

Antioxidants have a protective effect against free radicals which can damage DNA and cells. There are two types of antioxidants,

Bioenergetics is the study and process of how energy flows and how it is transformed.

Q10 is found to be lower in people with heart disease and diabetes.

Table showing types of antioxidant substances and their sources

Non enzymatic substances	Enzymatic sources	
Co enzyme Q10	Glutathione peroxidase	
Vitamin E	catalase	
Vitamin C		
carotenoids		
glutathione		
Lipoic acid		

Q10 is needed for proper glycaemic control and the prevention of endothelial dysfunction.

Endothelial dysfunction refers to the impaired functioning of the lining of blood vessels. It is characterised by poor vasodilation, a deficiency of nitric oxide (which dilates arteries and therefore lowers blood pressure), inflammation in the arteries (also known as an 'activated endothelium' with an enhanced risk of thrombosis (blood clotting).

It is a condition which precedes atherosclerosis but fortunately is reversible.

It is an independent risk factor for cardiovascular events.

Medical conditions that are associated with a Q10 deficiency are;

- Heart failure
- Coronary artery disease (CAD)
- Alzheimer's disease
- Motor neuron disease
- Cancer
- Chronic fatigue syndrom

Cholesterol is a type of lipid which is an essential structural component of animal cell membranes. It is therefore needed for the synthesis of new cells and the repair of cells

It has numerous applications in the body including:

- The synthesis of bile which helps to break down fats
- The synthesis of vitamin D from the sun's rays
- The synthesis of vital hormones
- The neutralisation of bacterial toxins
- The synthesis of immune cells required to beat infection
- It helps to regulate membrane fluidity over the range of physiological temperatures
- It helps to prevent anxiety and depression

To name but a few of its many and diverse functions.

The mass medication of populations with statins without sufficient reason to do so is extremely concerning.

Those individuals over the age of fifty-five, ethnic minorities which may be susceptible to diabetes or hypertension are routinely offered statins.

The impact of these actions may worsen the very conditions that statins were offered to an individual in the first place yet I have no confirmation of my many encounters with patients, that these side effects have ever been discussed with patients.

Cholesterol levels will rise and fall naturally and should be of no concern if it goes above an arbitrary level.

If you have an infection, then it is to be expected that cholesterol will rise. If you are stressed or need bile to digest food, then cholesterol levels will rise to accommodate these changes. This is all perfectly natural and does not need medicating.

The list of negative side effects from statins is appalling. Rhabdomyolyis – the sudden breakdown of muscle tissue which clogs kidneys and is fatal - is one such effect. Rare it may be but that is no comfort to the Tfamily of the person who has had it.

Maybe you would like 'visible fluid retention' or heart failure, constipation, diabetes, muscle aches, muscle inflammation – and remember the heart is a muscle - and memory loss are just a very small part of what statins can offer you. These are far more common.

The fact is that if statins are reducing your cholesterol they are blocking the MP and thus the other branches that should be synthesising vital key substances for the health of your body.

 You are informed that you will be on statins for life. What a clever trick to keep somebody - that doesn't need to be made this ill - providing profits for companies that make them. It is a high price to pay.

Indeed, it is concerning that when older people have been found to be healthier if their cholesterol levels are higher than our arbitrary figures, that we continue to feed them medication that will shorten their lives.

Does keeping to a low fat diet reduce cholesterol and the potential for heart attacks? Well, no. We have only to consider the French Paradox – high fat diets and low cardiovascular disease – or the Victorian diet, full of cream and butter and cheese, where diseases of the cardiovascular system weren't taught in medical school as there was simply no call for them.

Inflammation causes damaged arteries and an increased risk of cardiovascular damage. Saturated fats   do not initiate inflammatory processes. They do not have spare electrons, to do so, since by their very nature they are saturated.

Cholesterol does not cause inflammation but statins are known to. Cholesterol does not breakdown muscles and cells. It is a repairer and healing substance. Statins, however, do damage cells and tissues. So why are they prescribed in the numbers that they are?

We do know that sugar causes inflammation, accelerates aging and raises blood sugar levels so why do we continue to treat a condition for a cause that does not exist?

Inflammation

Just what is inflammation? That's probably a good question for many people. We have an idea when we see redness and swelling that inflammation is going on which will always be accompanied by pain. This pain can be diffuse especially when the source is inflammation occurring internally. The pain may also be referred pain so that it appears elsewhere than the original area of injury.

Researchers at the Medical College of Georgia discovered a nerve centre in a cell layer in the spleen that controls the immune response and therefore inflammation throughout the body. It is quelled by taking 2g of baking soda in water for two weeks.

The only downside to this is that this has the potential to raise your blood pressure. If you do have raised blood pressure hen taking 250mg of magnesium and a glass of tomato juice for the potassium will most likely address this.

Trace Elements and Metabolic Syndrome

Zinc

Zinc is a trace element which is often associated with the health of the immune system. Indeed, a zinc deficiency can lead to a vulnerability to infection. Zinc is better known for its ability to activate T lymphocytes. It also has a regulatory role in controlling the immune response as well as attacking cancerous and infected cell.   Zinc supplementation studies in the elderly have shown a reduction in the rate   and severity of infections, decreased   oxidative stress and the presence of fewer inflammatory cytokines.   However, its super status is not just confined to the health of the immune system.

Zinc is required for many functions in the body especially in relation to activating enzymes which speed up metabolic processes in the body.   Some of these processes may be related to wound healing and age-related chronic diseases such as age-related macular degeneration.   However, there are some quite remarkable effects on weight loss when a zinc deficiency is corrected. Since zinc deficiency is rife in society it is worth looking at the impact of zinc on weight and the underlying reasons why it might aid weight loss.

Zinc is essential for the smooth running of the thyroid gland. It is needed to produce thyroid stimulating hormone. The latter, if in short supply, results in low levels of T4 and T3. These hormones help regulate the body's metabolism turning food into energy. Without the proper synthesis of these hormones not only will weight gain occur but the person who lacks these thyroid hormones will feel cold and tired.

Zinc supplements help to increase the weight loss on those on a calorie restricted diets. In a study, calorie reduction of 300Kj was undertaken by individuals supplemented with 30mg of zinc. The control group did not receive any supplementary zinc. This regime was followed for 15 weeks. After 15 weeks there was a significant reduction of body weight, BMI, waist circumference in the zinc supplemented group. In addition, it was found that there were lower levels of C-reactive protein, insulin resistance and appetite score.

Therefore, zinc appears to tackle obesity from different angles. Firstly, it helps correct any deficiency which might impact the metabolic rate. Secondly, it tackles insulin resistance enabling food to be used as an energy source instead of being used for fat storage. Thirdly, it aids appetite reduction and fourthly it helps tackle inflammation.

Many comorbid conditions occur alongside obesity and metabolic syndrome. They are all associated with zinc deficiency. There are a number of skin reactions, including psoriasis, that may be due to insufficient zinc in the diet. Delayed wound healing, decline of reproductive capacity, mental lethargy, depression, and susceptibility to Alzheimer's Disease are also included.

Oxidative stress underlies the molecular mechanisms responsible for the development of many inflammatory diseases like atherosclerosis, diabetes mellitus, rheumatoid arthritis as well as neurodegenerative disorders. The cellular antioxidant system proves insufficient to remove the reactive oxygen species which damage cells and create inflammation in this process.

The regulatory function of zinc cannot be underestimated. It is essential to the structure and function of nearly 3000 macromolecules and over 300 enzymes.

Macromolecules are very large molecules such as proteins made from amino acids.

Common macromolecules, monomers and some end products are:

MACROMOLECULE	MONOMERS (the building blocks)	END PRODUCT
protein	Amino acids	Protein – many types such as keratin for hair and collagen for connective tissue, enzymes and antibodies.
Nucleic acids	Nucleotides	RNA and DNA
Lipids	Fatty acids	Fats, sterols, waxes and oils

Although Zinc is known for its antiviral impact, it also has a beneficial effect on secretory molecules and the bactericidal activity of human peptidoglycan recognition proteins. (PGLYRP's)

Peptidoglycan is a substance that forms the cell walls of bacteria. The ability of the immune system to detect bacteria – and thus deal with it – is partially dependent on the available serum zinc.

The importance of having adequate daily amounts of zinc cannot be underestimated. Zinc has been described as the element with a minor plasma pool and a rapid turnover.

There are certain groups of individuals that are more susceptible to zinc deficiency. These include:

- Diabetics
- Cancer patients
- Those with liver disease
- Those on a high plant diet as the phytates in plants bind to zinc
- Those on high copper or high iron diets
- Those who are on a calorie reducing diet
- Those who are under stress
- The elderly
- Breast fed babies
- Pregnant women
- Alcoholism
- Those with malabsorption problems of the digestive tract such as Crohn's disease.

Sources of zinc include:

- Oysters (very high in zinc) 3 ounces provides 673% of the daily value
- Beef – 3 ounces provide 65% of your daily requirements
- Beef patty – 3 ounces provides 64% of your daily requirement
- Baked beans – half a cup provides 26% of your daily requirement.

The benefits of zinc for metabolic syndrome and its related comorbidities cannot be understated.

The Daily Requirement of Zinc has been placed at'

Men – 11g

Women 8mg

However, for short periods of no greater than a month, upwards of this amount may be used to aid the processes which counteract metabolic syndrome. Any longer and you raise the risk of iron and copper depletion which carry their own risk of deficiency diseases.

Boron

Boron is a trace mineral that has many important functions in the body that are relevant to metabolic syndrome. While boron is generally associated with the health of bone it is essential for wound healing which is often delayed in those with metabolic syndrome.

Further, boron is required for the optimum use of hormones such as oestrogen and testosterone. It is able to increase oestrogen in post-menopausal women and healthy men. Oestrogen is important when looking at potential reasons for weight gain because low levels may contribute to abdominal weight gain.

Boron enhances magnesium and vitamin D absorption and also helps reduce inflammatory markers such as C-reactive protein and tumour necrosis factor (TNF-α).

C-reactive protein is a substance produced by the liver in response to inflammation. The blood test for C-reactive protein is a common one. While it tests for levels of inflammation it cannot indicate the cause of the inflammation. However, as inflammation is rife in those with metabolic syndrome, it is a good test in that it alerts you to this underlying problem and the need to address it.

TNF-α is also a marker of inflammation. It helps to coordinate the inflammatory process. Sometimes TNF may get out of control. When it does symptoms may include:

- Low blood pressure

- Loss of appetite

- Redness and swelling at the site of injury

- Fever and muscle aches and pains

There is also an association between TNF-α and insulin resistance responsible for diabetes type. It is a bit of a catch 22 situation because insulin resistance leads to obesity and obesity promotes the generation of more TNF-α   which in turn leads to greater insulin resistance. TNF is released by many cells including:

- Macrophages

- T cells

- Fibroblasts

- Dendritic cells

- Fat cells

In particular, TNF is highly likely to affect cells that line blood vessels creating inflammation and laying down an environment for plaques which block blood flow.

Vascular problems that ensue cause angiogenesis which is found in conditions like lymphoedema and cancer.

TNF may also be responsible for intestinal problems such as irritable bowel syndrome and the inflammatory bowel diseases such as Crohn's disease. It does this by stimulating effector T cells and macrophages. When these cells are stimulated they produce more inflammatory substances and resist programmed cell death, a process known as apoptosis. Apoptosis is required to eliminate cancerous cells.

There are many factors that increase TNF and these include but are not limited to:

- A lack of exercise but **excessive** exercise would increase TNF.

- Obesity

- High glucose levels

- A high fat diet

- Smoking and alcohol

- Deficiencies of choline, magnesium, zinc, chromium and vitamin D.

Finally, boron has a suppressive role on adiopogenic differentiation. What does this mean? Basically, pre fat cells develop into mature ones during this process of differentiation and is to be avoided if we are serious about losing weight.

Boron can be taken up to 20mg daily but the normal supplemented dose is 3 mg. it is better to keep to the lower end of the dosage recommendations if you are using it just as a preventative. Boron, in high doses, can actually cause weight gain and hair loss. In smaller doses its main function appears to be optimising the function of other vital nutrients.

Good sources of boron are:

- Dried beans

- Milk

- Potatoes

- Coffee

- Apples

- Brazil nuts

Quercetin

In this chapter the impact of quercetin on many conditions is covered, not just metabolic syndrome. This is because metabolic syndrome will not exist in isolation from many other diseases whose roots are firmly found in chronic inflammation.

Quercetin is a natural pigment or flavonoid which is found in many fruits, vegetables and grains as well as wine and tea. Red onions are particularly rich in quercetin. It has antioxidant properties and these properties help combat the damaging effects of free radicals.

Free radicals are unpaired electrons. These free radicals are the cause of chronic disease which is so rife in society. Antioxidants are able to bind to free radicals and neutralise them in the process. This stops the chronic inflammatory processes which are associated with many diseases including diabetes, lymphoedema, lipoedema, arthritis, high blood pressure and many neurodegenerative disorders. This is not a definitive list.

It is often observed that individuals do not just suffer from one inflammatory disorder but a whole plethora of them. In metabolic syndrome the risks of cardiovascular disease, stroke and diabetes are well known but alongside that it is not unusual to find that the diabetic has osteoarthritis or other inflammatory conditions. I have certainly found it to be useful in rosacea and psoriasis.

Quercetin is also useful in conditions where there is an allergy involved such as hay fever and angieoedema. Research has shown that in peanut related anaphylaxis, quercetin completely prevented the need for medication when taken at 500mg daily.

Quercetin's benefits do not stop their either though. It has anti-tumour activity.   Its properties inhibit the proliferation of cancer cells by inducing apoptosis (cell death) as well as arresting the cell cycle of cancers.

If this wasn't enough, quercetin has anti-fibrotic activity and is particularly useful for those with radiation fibrosis, and the fibrosis that occurs in lymphoedema and lipoedema due to inflamed subcutaneous tissue.

Inflammation can cause an increase in blood pressure which is a major contributor of heart disease. Inflammation generally follows metabolic disturbance seen in abnormalities such as diabetes, dyslipoedema, obesity, insulin resistance and hyperinsulinemia. The ensuing inflammation leads to a rise in arterial blood pressure.

Brown fat, white fat – what's serotonin got to do with it?

All fat is not equal when it comes to burning calories. The fact that fat burns any calories may come as a surprise to some. After all, we can understand that we store fat but not that it burns calories but while white fat builds up in obesity, brown fat produces an important protein that helps to promote energy to generate heat. Therefore, it seems wise to take a closer look at these two types of fat.

White fat is found in the subcutaneous region, that is just under the skin. It provides the padding we need so that we do not injure ourselves and also provides insulation in cold weather. This type of fat is also the visceral fat, found around organs which pumps out inflammatory chemicals and is likely to raise your blood pressure as well as deposit itself in that well known apple shape found in metabolic syndrome.

Brown fat is found in deposits around the kidneys, along the spinal cord and between the shoulder blades. It consists of many lipid droplets. There is far less brown fat than white fat in obese people   and brown fat does not build up in obese people.

Research has shown that white fat is linked with certain branched chain and aromatic amino acids.

The branched chain amino acids are:

- Leucine
- Isoleucine
- Valine

The aromatic amino acids are:

- Phenylalanine
- Tyrosine

These amino acids when eaten have been closely related to type 2 diabetes, insulin resistance, obesity and future diabetes.

As these amino acids are so important to the progression of diabetes the main sources of these are tabulated below.

Table showing the amino acids associated with obesity and their main sources

Amino acids	Food sources
Leucine	Dairy, soy, beans and legumes
Isoleucine	Beef, chicken, pork, tuna, dairy, lentils and beans[12]
Valine	Soy, cheese, peanuts, mushrooms, whole grains, vegetables
Phenylalanine	Dairy, meat, poultry, soy, beans, nuts and fish
tyrosine	Poultry, fish, peanuts, nuts, bananas, dairy, lima beans pumpkin and sesame seeds

Now as you can see most of the foods that can contribute to obesity are the high protein foods – those very foods you are told to eat because if you keep up the high protein foods and cut out fat/and or/ carbohydrates then you will lose weight.

---

[12] https://www.myfooddata.com/articles/high-isoleucine-foods.php#isoleucine-food-list

This may happen for some individuals but others will just find that they want to binge on something sweet when they are on a high protein, low carbohydrate/fat diet.

There is real science why this is so and why many people on a high protein diet cannot lose weight. It is all to do with brown fat

Brown fat produces a protein called SLC25A44 which for simplicity sake I am just going to call brown fat protein. It has a special function in that it brings the branched chain amino acids into the mitochondria, where they are used to provide energy and generate heat. When this process is blocked, studies in mice have shown that higher serum levels of branched chain amino acids result in obesity and signs of diabetes.

The lack of serotonin blocks this process for serotonin enhances the function of brown fat which is to break down blood sugar and fat molecules.

Serotonin is found in carbohydrates and sugary foods. Its parent amino acid is tryptophan an amino acid which has the largest molecules of any amino acid.

When it tries to compete with other amino acids to cross the blood brain barrier, it gets left behind. It really needs a little carbohydrate to help it to accomplish this task.

Tryptophan can follow one of two pathways. It can go down the kyurenic acid pathway. Kyurenic acid inhibits colon cancer proliferation or it can become part of central serotonin which increases energy expenditure by enhancing the sympathetic drive to brown adipose tissue.

Serotonin is the happiness hormone. It stops you feeling anxious and depressed. It can be seen that too little carbohydrate to protein in the diet just promotes a build-up of branched chain amino acids leading to obesity, diabetes and metabolic syndrome.

Tryptophan requires the enzyme tryptophan hydroxylase to convert it to serotonin.

This enzyme is dependent on oxygen and a substance called tetrahydrobiopterin for regulation. Therefore, they are cofactors and vital for the conversion of tryptophan to its intermediate – 5 htp – to serotonin.

Nutrients which support the production of tetrahydrobiopterin are:

- Vitamin C
- Curcumin
- Methyl folate

Vitamin C is found in fresh fruit and vegetables. It is a water soluble vitamin and cannot be stored in the body as the fat soluble vitamins A, D, E and K can, therefore it is better that fresh fruit and vegetables are eaten every day. It is easily destroyed by sunlight and heat so cook any vegetables lightly.

 Curcumin is a bright yellow compound produced by the Curcuma longa plant found in turmeric which is used in curries. It is better known as a natural compound which has anti-viral activity. Investigations showed that it had efficacy against influenza A as well as a wide range of other.

Methyl folate is the active form of folic acid. It is also referred to as vitamin B9. This is an important vitamin which aids the conversion of homocysteine (a harmful amino acid) back into the harmless methionine.

 There are many good sources of methyl folate which include:

- Dark green leafy vegetables especially spinach and Brussels sprouts.
- liver
- Fruit
- Legumes
- Seafood
- Eggs
- Dairy products
- Meat
- grains

Many people who have been on a high protein diet for a long time and have failed to lose weight should try supplementing their diet with tryptophan 500mg –or 5htp - which is obtainable as a supplement (must be taken without other forms of protein but with a little carbohydrate for it to be absorbed). Alternatively, they could try substituting some of their protein for a little carbohydrate.

In a nutshell

SEROTONIN PERSUADES BROWN FAT TO BURN UP THE AMINO ACIDS WHICH CONTRIBUTE TO OBESITY, METABOLIC SYNDROME AND DIABETES

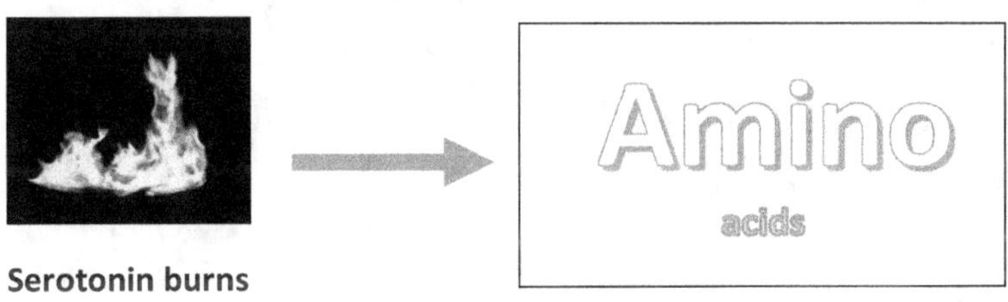

Serotonin burns

SEROTONIN IS FORMED FROM TRYPTOPHAN WHICH IS A LARGE AMINO ACID.

TRYPTOPHAN IS SO BIG UNABLE TO COMPETE WITH OTHER SMALLER AMINO ACIDS TO CROSS THE BLOOD

BRAIN BARRIER ON A TRANSPORTER. THEREFORE, IT IS BETTER TO BE TAKEN BY ITSELF WITH A LITTLE CARBOHYDRATE.

Or

YOU CAN SUPPLEMENT WITH 5HTP WHICH IS THE INTERMEDIARY PRODUCT FORMED OF TRYPTOPHAN AND SEROTONIN.

Tryptophan is found in most **high**-protein **foods**, including wheat germ, cottage cheese, chicken, and turkey.

We have now completed the chapter on fats and serotonin but there is yet another exciting substance which must be included in this book. It holds a great deal of promise for those with metabolic syndrome as it has anti-inflammatory and fat burning qualities.

Carvacrol –prevents the formation of fat cells (as do indoles)

No chapter of any book connected with obesity, fat storage, metabolic syndrome, lipoedema would be complete without a chapter on carvacrol. It has numerous properties including being a natural antibiotic, an antimicrobial in general, an anti-inflammatory and analgesic. However, it also prevents adipogenesis. This means that it prevents the creation of new fat cells especially in those people who eat a high fat diet. So what exactly is carvacrol?

Carvacrol is a substance found in aromatic plants like oregano, thyme and wild bergamot. It is mildly acidic.

There are a number of foods which contain free and bound phenol compounds.

 Bound phenolic compounds are especially found in cereals. They are important antioxidants. In addition, they inhibit cancerous cell growth and impact on important enzymes which are involved in the metabolism of carbohydrates.

Both free and bound phenols are found in foods such as:

- Peanuts
- Oranges, apples, bananas, red grapes, tomatoes and other highly coloured fruits
- Cocoa

- Milk

Salicylates which are found in aspirin (as a non-food substance) also contain phenols.

Now this is all very interesting but it is the conditions where adipogenesis impacts that makes carvacrol so interesting.

A study undertaken by Cho et al was entitled *Carvacrol prevents diet-induced obesity by modulating gene expressions involved in adipogenesis and inflammation in mice fed with high-fat diet.*

It was published in the Journal of Nutritional Biochemistry.

A high fat diet was fed to male mice with the intention of investigating the underlying mechanisms of gene expression which are involved in the production of heat, fat cells and inflammation.

The mice were divided into 3 groups.

1. Normal diet
2. High fat diet
3. Diet supplemented with carvacrol at 0.1%

Various features were measured including body weight. In addition, adipose tissue genes were also assessed.

The results showed that the mice fed with the added carvacrol had a 'significantly reduced body weight gain'.

It was found that the carvacrol diet significantly reversed the processes that led to the creation of fat cells and inflammation. Further, it lowered plasma lipid levels

Excitingly, the fat that was inhibited was the visceral fat which packs itself around organs and pumps out inflammatory cytokines (chemicals).

The study suggest that it was able to do this through a number of pathways including:

- Suppressing bone morphogenic protein – fibroblast growth factor 1
- Galanin- mediated signaling,
- Attenuating the production of inflammation causing chemicals in visceral adipose tissue through inhibiting two receptors (TLR2 and TLR-4) mediated signalling.

Although carvacrol has rapid and significant results (I have experienced these myself) there are many other food sources which help to modulate multiple genes which aid lipogenesis. We turn to these now.

Diet induced obesity prevented by indole-3 carbinol

Indole-3 carbinol is produced by the breakdown of a substance called glucosinolate glucobrassion. It is found in good amounts in cruciferous vegetables which include:

- Brussels sprouts
- Broccoli
- Kale
- Cabbage
- Cauliflower
- Collard green

Many people juice these to produce a pleasant tasting drink high in the active ingredient we are require.

In a similar study to the one involving carvacrol mice were assigned to receive either a normal, high fat or a diet supplemented with indole-3 carbinol at 1g per kilogram of body weight.

This substance worked in a number of ways to reduce weight including:

- Regulating receptors which normalise weight which were down regulated during high fat diets.
- Decreasing expression of some adiopogenic factors
- Ameliorating the expression of inflammatory cytokines
- Increasing thermogenesis

Therefore, it appears overall that there is decreased creation of fat cell and inflammation and thermogenesis was activated.

Epigallocatechin-3-gallate

This is a substance that is found in green tea and helps to regulate multiple genes which are expressed in fat tissue of obese mice where the obesity is due to diet.

The results were similar to those found in the above two studies. Weight loss occurred and was likely due to regulation of genes in white adipose tissue as well as increased thermogenesis.

Others substances which have similar effects are chit oligosaccharide with its main effects through reducing gene expression in adipogenesis and through the reduction of inflammation.   This substance is found in prawns and the shells of sea creatures like crabs.

Resveratrol

Phytochemicals – chemicals which are derived from plants- have many uses when it comes to regulating weight gain. They inhibit the differentiation of pre-adipocytes thus preventing the maturation of fat cells.

In addition, they encourage the breakdown of fat cells to be used as energy and induce apoptosis of existing adipocytes thus reducing fat mass.

Resveratrol also decreases the creation of fat cells through a number of mechanisms. Further, it increases lipolysis but, it should be born in mind that most of these weight reductions are for those on high fat diets. Whether weight reduction would occur in those with high carbohydrate diets is not known.

This study was extended to include quercetin, vitamin D and Genistein and this combination not only decreased weight gain but was found to inhibit bone loss, too.

It appears that combinations of phytochemicals have even greater impact on the mechanisms that cause obesity and can effectively prevent weight gain and induce weight loss.

There are many different groups of phytochemicals. They all have different chemical structures. As they are metabolised differently, they may have different functions on health. This is why the general advice is to eat as wide a range of colours in fruits and vegetables as possible.

Some examples of phytonutrients can be found below.

Table showing examples of phytonutrients and their food sources.

Phytonutrient	Food sources
Flavonoids like quercetin and anthocyanins	Soybeans, onions, apples, tea, coffee
Carotenoids like lycopene, lutein, beta carotene, zeaxanthin	Found in orange, red and dark green foods like carrots, tomatoes and dark green leafy veg
Polyphenols like resveratrol and ellagic acid	Red grapes and wine, berries, green tea and whole grains
tannins	Cereals, beans nuts, wine cocoa
curcuminoids	Curcumin from turmeric
Carvacrol	Oregano, thyme, wild bergamot

A study on an obese 65-year-old female using 500mg of tryptophan and 50mg of oregano oil.

The subject had long term weight problems which had proved resistant to a calorie reduced diet with increased exercise. The latter consisted of walking an extra mile every day with some intermittent gym activity when it could be fitted in.

The subject restricted her diet to 1500 calories daily and did not depart from this.

After two weeks the subject had not lost any weight whatsoever. She reduced this to 1250 for a further two weeks. After two weeks she had still not lost any weight and was finding it hard to maintain the exercise regime and did not want to stick to such a low calorie diet.

It was agreed that she would take 500mg of tryptophan and 50mg of oregano oil daily while taking her normal meals. She was advised to take the tryptophan away from the main meal and take it with a little carbohydrate such as half a biscuit.

 She would record her weight daily, in the morning.

The results are tabulated below.

Table showing weight changes in a 65-year-old woman after taking supplements of 500mg of tryptophan and 50mg of oregano oil   while continuing to eat her normal diet

Day	Amount of loss or gain
1-3	No loss or gain
4	1.2lb
5	1lb
6	1/2lb
7	No change
8	1/2lb

 The overall weight loss over a period of 8 days was 3.2lb

Since the cause of weight gain can differ amongst individuals, there is no guarantee of success with this combination of food supplements. Nevertheless, carvacrol can produce rapid fat burning, a lowering of inflammation and a reduction in risk infection - which help to reduce the changes that are found in metabolic syndrome – in some people who have found it difficult to lose weight.

The Role of Potassium in Weight Loss

While most studies focus on calorie reduction of carbohydrates and fat to reduce the impact of metabolic syndrome, more recent studies[13] have looked at the impact of electrolytes in this process. In particular, increments in dietary potassium has been found to predict weight loss during treatment of metabolic syndrome and obesity.

Potassium has not generally been seen as a major contributor in responding to metabolic syndrome. Most people have heard of potassium but there has been little in the media to suggest that there is a deficiency of this mineral cum electrolyte in the population as a whole.

 However, potassium is a vital mineral and an electrolyte. It is essential for enabling your muscles to work effectively. This also includes muscles like your heart and the ones that control breathing. Individuals with low potassium levels often have digestive problems like slow bowel transit which may result in constipation and impaction. Just walking may be

---

13

https://www.ncbi.nlm.nih.gov/pmc/articles/PMC6627830/#:~:text=It%20is%20notable%20that%20the,and%20in%20overall%20calori c%20intake.

problematical; legs may feel heavy and taking steps an effort. Brain fog and the inability to remember recent events may also be due to low potassium levels.

The importance of potassium in lymphoedema – which often occurs alongside metabolic syndrome – cannot be underplayed either. Unlike the circulatory system, which does have a pump to enable blood to be distributed around the body – the lymphatic system does not. However, the potassium channels are vital to lymph pump activity, formation and its transportation. Without adequate potassium, lymphatic fluid is hampered and may account for the development of secondary lymphoedema.

As lymphoedema and lipoedema often occur alongside each other, then improving potassium intake in cases of deficiency for lipoedema may also help ameliorate this condition.

There have been a number of studies that have shown an association between lymphoedema and some lung problems. When it affects the head and neck this generally occurs at the same time as any external swelling. Changes in voice quality may occur. The voice may be more   raspy, singers may not be able to reach the notes that they could do. Difficulty in swallowing or a sense of something stuck in the back of the throat often occurs. This often leads to people swallowing air in an effort to dislodge whatever is stuck in the back of the throat. Breathing may become more laboured.

Diuretics are frowned upon if you have lymphoedema purely because when fluid is lost then lymph becomes thicker and does not flow as easily. The importance of the pumping action required to move lymph has not gained as much publicity.   The connection between metabolic syndrome, low potassium levels, abdominal obesity and lymphoedema does not appear to have been given the importance that it deserves in research. There is very little of this nature to be found.

A number of medications can cause low potassium levels. (hypokalaemia) Most notably the non-potassium sparing diuretics   like Furosemide while ridding the body of excess fluid also carry with it important minerals like potassium and magnesium. Insulin also causes more potassium to be removed from the blood to cells and can result in a temporary hypokalaemia. Ace inhibitors and non-steroidal anti-inflammatory drugs also have the capacity to raise potassium levels.

There are also potassium sparing diuretics which have the potential to raise potassium levels.

Low potassium levels are associated with low magnesium levels. Magnesium is one of the minerals lost during diuretic use. In addition, many studies show that a greater percentage of the population are deficient in magnesium due to poor diets. The impact of poor nutrition and the side effects of diuretic medication have the ability to cause poor health.

Magnesium is a cofactor in more than 300 enzyme systems. These systems regulate a diversity of biochemical reactions in the body. These include blood glucose control, protein synthesis, blood pressure regulation, among many others. In relation to potassium, it has a role to play in actively transporting calcium and potassium ions across cell membranes. This is necessary for normal heart rhythm, muscle contraction and the conduction of nerve impulses.

The concept of prescribing diuretics to reduce blood pressure is a peculiar one. Low potassium levels will raise your blood pressure as well as giving a propensity to a pot belly. Low potassium levels also encourage the build-up of visceral fat which pumps out inflammatory chemicals.

In the study referred to above, the first 68 participants aged between 18 and 70 years completed a full year's intervention. During this time, they were expected to complete 150 minutes of exercise weekly. In addition, calories were restricted by 25-30% of the normal metabolic resting rate.

The participants were seen by a nutritionist and a physician on a regular basis. The differences were examined after one year.

In that year, participants lost on average 9.36kg. This represented up to a 16.4% reduction in body mass index. Analysis revealed that the percentage change was related to the consumption of potassium, vitamin B6, caporic acid, calcium, sugars and total energy consumption.   However, the increase in potassium intake was the strongest indicator of reduction of the BMI closely followed by caproic acid (found in goat's milk).

The range within which potassium works without problems is narrow but any excess is cleared away by the kidneys providing, of course, that the kidneys are functioning correctly.

The Dietary Recommended Intake of potassium is not reached by most people in Western countries. The study showed that the average daily potassium intake in adults was 2.9 - 3.2 for men (DRI is 4.7g. In women this was found to be even less at 2.1-2.3g. Taking this further, the findings were that only 10% of men and only 1% of women were reaching their DRI of potassium.

It has been suggested that low potassium levels are unlikely to be caused by poor dietary habits. The reasoning behind this is that many foods contain potassium including:

- Dark leafy greens
- Potatoes
- Bananas
- Fish
- beans

Bananas particularly are advertised as a good source of potassium and they are but they still only provide one tenth of our daily potassium needs. Potatoes, once found on a daily basis in various forms on our plates have now been replaced with rice, pasta and other grains.

Our diets have changed over the years and, as such, the nutrients we ingest have changed. These changes bring new health conditions with them while others will shuffle away.

In addition, when calorie reduction is undertaken, it is highly likely that   there is a reduction in the intake of food and food choices. The knock on effect of this is that potassium intake is likely to be reduced as well.

Calorie reduction may then not aid weight loss leading to a frustrating and fruitless attempt to lose weight before any thoughts of dietary responses to health conditions are abandoned altogether.

Potassium supplementation is not generally recommended because it is only safe within narrow limits. For this reason, supplements are only found in 99mg doses.   Generally, up to 4 daily are recommended but this amount is often less than you would find in one banana. GP's may prescribe higher doses but this generally after tests for suspected potassium deficiency.

Home tests are not available for potassium deficiency.

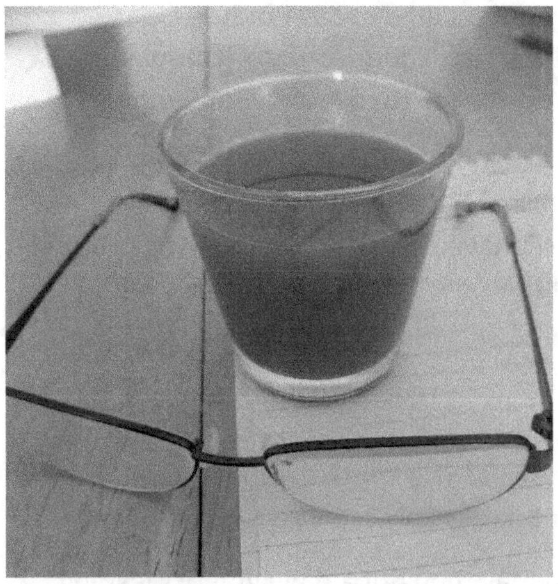

Tomato juice contains good amounts of potassium

Some foods which contain reasonable amounts of potassium are:

food	Amount of potassium
Decaffeinated expresso coffee	One cup of prepared coffee 116mg
Low sodium baking powder	560mg
Tomato juice l00mg	229 mg in
Banana l00g	358mg
I cup of strong black tea	90mg
Potato 100g	421 mg
Spinach - one cupful – approx. 30mg	170mg
Milk 240g	366mg
Mushroom 100g	318mg
Cucumber one cup	200mg of potassium
Melon 100g	270mg
Nectarine 100g	200mg
Dates 100mg	656 mg
Dried apricots 100mg	1162mg
Baked beans100mg	358mg

- note: one 1000mg is equal to one g
- one ml is equal to one mg

A useful link for those wishing to increase their potassium intake can be found here.

https://louisville.edu/medicine/departments/familymedicine/files/Potassium%20Food%20List.pdf

However, from the above it should be clear that it is not always that easy to take in the DRI of potassium especially for those who do not have well planned and diverse diets and are restricting calories too.

It is clearly important to remember that without adequate magnesium, potassium – no matter how much you ingested – would simply not be available to the body.

The study found that 37 subjects increase their potassium and 27 decreased this mineral. After one year it was found that those who increased their potassium had a greater weight loss than those who decreased their ingestion of potassium during calorie restriction.

It is always a useful exercise to jot down your food intake over a period of 3 days to ascertain if your diet does contain enough potassium and magnesium.

They are important nutrients for the prevention of a host of other medical ailments including high blood pressure and stroke.

Other books by this author include:

- The EDS and Hypermobility Syndrome Diet
- Alleviating Symptoms of EDS
- Gastroparesis
- The EDS recipe book
- The Lipoedema Diet
- The Lymphoedema Diet: reverse and repair lymphatic damage
- The Anti Virus Diet
- The Asthma Diet
- The Reluctant Bowel
- The MND Diet
- Why we live longer with higher cholesterol levels
- A dietary connection for MACS, POTS and EDS
- Identity: a self-exploration workbook *
- Journey Through Pneumonia
- https://www.amazon.co.uk/dp/B07TBHMV6N

*This book can be used alone or in small group work and is an excellent resource for those who are 'people helpers.'

Among many others

They are available on Amazon

Lynne has written a semi-autobiographical trilogy.

** While this trilogy is available on kindle and paperback on Amazon, it may be cheaper to buy from the link below.**

They may be obtained off the publisher's website, in paperback form, where they are more reasonably priced.

https://www.shieldcrest.co.uk/?s=lynne+d+m+noble++

For the full range of books by this author, visit the author website on

https://www.amazon.co.uk/-/e/B07BPQZ5CD

https://www.amazon.com/-/e/B07BPQZ5CD

A percentage of the profits from the sale of these books go to support charities like the Exodus Project below.

The Exodus Project

My first introduction to the far reaching impact of The Exodus Project occurred when I was travelling around Cawthorne in one of their buses, visiting gardens.   A young lad was happily munching on a sandwich. He looked up briefly, pointed to the driver and said,' He's my second dad, he is,' then he returned to his sandwich without further comment

Such remarks are often very telling and so I arranged to meet Jackie Peel and Martin Sawdon, at the charity's premises in Barnsley. They set up the Exodus Project 20 years ago. They moved into their current premises – a redundant Methodist church - in 2010.

Both Jackie and Martin have been youth workers in their church. Martin worked in housing for the homeless in addition to working in learning disabilities services in institutional settings.

The work that the Exodus Project undertakes is of paramount importance to the communities it serves. These were former mining communities which became disadvantaged after pit-closures. Currently about 400 children attend mid-week activities from Monday to Thursday inclusive. These activities include dance, drama, craft, music, sports and games. In addition, there are weekend camps, cycle treks, outward bound activities, bowling and swimming. The children are taught valuable life skills including how to cook and   bake. It is all about teaching children how to fulfil their potential and learn skills they will be able to pass onto the next generation.

The grounds, once overgrown, have been turned into   a play- and camping - ground. A miniature railway is in the process of being installed.

Martin and Jackie have developed a unique model in that The Exodus Project goes beyond dispensing services. They are keen to build up relationships with the whole family and not just the child that attends the mid- week clubs. In addition, once children have reached the age of fourteen, they are invited to help out with the younger groups as junior volunteers. Once they reach the age of eighteen, they become adult volunteers. This model provides a constant supply of help from individuals who have   benefitted already from attending such groups.

The building is large and inviting. It is decorated with bold colours and has comfy seating. It is a real home from home; a haven for families who have been disadvantaged by the closure of the life force of its community.

Martin and Jackie have clear ideas about how they wish to develop the Exodus Project but the lottery funding which they benefitted from is no longer available. Sadly, they have had to close two of their clubs due to lack of funding. This decision wasn't taken lightly. They do have two charity shops which raises some money and they obtain some funding from outside organisations for the use of their facilities. However, this is clearly not enough to keep their clubs, weekend activities and building going to cater for the ever growing number of children who are benefitting from the work being undertaken here.   Neither does it allow for future development.

Exodus do have a Just Giving page which can be found here if you wish to help further their work https://www.justgiving.com/exodus

In addition, you can keep up with activities on their Facebook page here

https://www.facebook.com/search/top/?q=the%20exodus%20project%20barnsley&epa=SEARCH_BOX

Lynne's blog and twitter posts can be found here:

https://quintessentiallylynne.weebly.com/nutritional-medicine.html

twitter: Lynne D M Noble@ldmn53